# FOOD NOISE

# FOOD
# N◀))OISE

How weight loss medications & smart
nutrition can silence your cravings

# DR JACK MOSLEY

Foreword by Dr Clare Bailey Mosley

First published in Great Britain in 2025 by Short Books,
an imprint of wPublishing Group Ltd
Carmelite House
50 Victoria Embankment
London EC4Y 0DZ
www.octopusbooks.co.uk
www.octopusbooksusa.com

An Hachette UK Company
www.hachette.co.uk

The authorized representative in the EEA is Hachette Ireland, 8 Castlecourt Centre,
Dublin 15, D15 XTP3, Ireland (email: info@hbgi.ie)

Distributed in the US by Hachette Book Group, 1290 Avenue of the Americas,
4th and 5th Floors, New York, NY 10104

Distributed in Canada by Canadian Manda Group, 664 Annette Street, Toronto, Ontario, Canada M6S 2C8

ISBN 978-1-80419-334-1

A CIP catalogue record for this book is available from the British Library.

Typeset in 13/20pt Garamond Premier Pro by Jouve (UK), Milton Keynes.

Printed and bound in Great Britain by Clays Ltd, Elcograf S.p.A.

13579108642

Publisher: Jo Morrell
Commissioning Editor: Katie Forsythe
Creative Director: Mel Four
Senior Editor: Leanne Bryan
Copy Editor: Jo Roberts-Miller
Production Controller: Sarah Parry

This FSC®label means that materials used for the product have been responsibly sourced.

**Disclaimer**
All reasonable care has been taken in the preparation of this book but the information it contains is not
intended to take the place treatment by a qualified medical practitioner.

Before making any changes in your health regime, always consult a doctor. While all the therapies detailed
in this book are completely safe if done correctly, you must seek professional advice if you are in any
doubt about any medical condition. Any application of the ideas and information contained in
this book is at the reader's sole discretion and risk.

*I'd like to dedicate this book to my Dad, Michael Mosley.*
*He was a guiding light to my siblings and me, and an incredible,*
*warm, fun, caring father and husband. We all miss you.*

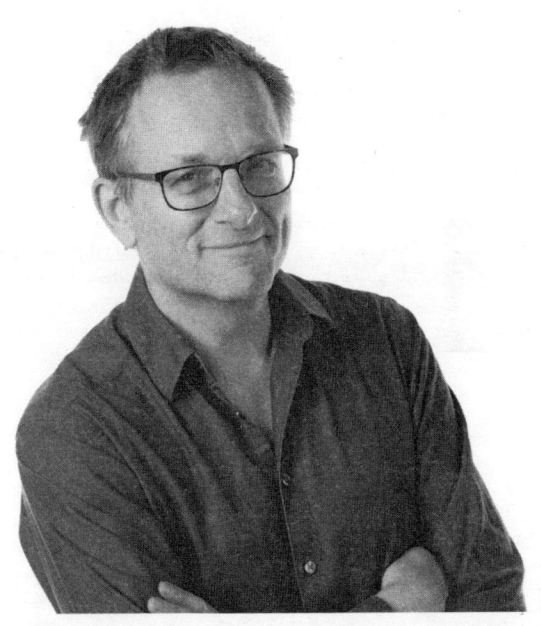

**Dr Michael Mosley** (1957–2024) was a much-loved author,
journalist, podcast host and television presenter. Michael
pioneered the Fast 800 programme, which helped countless people
improve their health, particularly those with type 2 diabetes.
His bestselling books include *The Fast Diet*, *The 8-Week Blood
Sugar Diet*, *The Clever Guts Diet*, *The Fast 800*, *The Fast 800 Keto*,
*Just One Thing* and *4 Weeks to Better Sleep*. He and his wife,
Dr Clare Bailey Mosley, have four children.

# CONTENTS

This introduction has a bittersweet flavour, following the terrible loss of my lovely husband Michael Mosley in Greece on the hottest day for decades. But the family and I have been able to get some consolation seeing my son Jack, a doctor, truly step up to the plate to write this informative and timely book.

For some time, Michael had been following the extraordinary explosion of the weight loss drugs with fascination. He could see clearly that they were a game changer, enabling people to shed significant amounts of weight. He could see the significant potential benefits, but he was also well aware that they are powerful and need to be used with some degree of support, and alongside a good-quality lifestyle programme.

But these new medications have also created a 'Wild West' out there, with minimal or no regulation or support. We are now scrambling to make sense of how these drugs will change the weight loss environment – for better or worse.

It wasn't until Jack and I were having a conversation about how transformative the weight loss medications are, when it comes to shedding the pounds, that it became obvious he should write about this weight loss revolution. Drawing on Jack's work as a GP registrar and his Master of Research in diabetes, as well as occasional support from me and the team at The Fast 800 programme, he felt he could bring some clarity to this fast-moving area of weight loss.

This exciting new frontier had opened up opportunities for weight loss which we could previously only have dreamt. Inevitably, there are potential side effects and risks to deal with, too. So, on a packed train from Austria, sharing a seat, we drew up the chapter headings. Jack's medical knowledge and passion to help others (just like his father) means he is the ideal person to write this book.

It is clear that suitable support programmes, such as The Fast 800 (www.thefast800.com), and the *Fast 800 Keto Recipe Book*, could also be part of the solution. At the back of this book, you will find nutritious recipes containing plenty of satiating protein and fibre (that also fit with the Fast 800 plan) and are suited to rapid weight loss and maintenance.

Jack has stepped into some big shoes, and I couldn't be more proud.

Clare Mosley, January 2025

# INTRODUCTION

My dad, Michael Mosley, was an inspiration to millions of people worldwide – particularly those living with obesity or type 2 diabetes. In the afternoon of 5 June 2024 he suddenly disappeared on the beautiful Greek island of Symi. His disappearance and death came as a huge shock to my mother, my siblings, myself and dad's family and friends, but also to many people around the world. He was such a likeable, relatable, familiar face that many felt they had lost a friend.

Dad's passion was medicine, science and changing people's lives. He was originally inspired to focus on diet after seeing his own father Bill's health decline. Bill had a terrible sweet tooth and he suffered from a number of weight-related diseases, including type 2 diabetes, osteoarthritis in his knees, high blood pressure, coronary heart disease and, eventually, mild dementia. Bill made many attempts to improve his diet, including trying The Cabbage Soup Diet and toasting a slice of organic wholegrain bread for breakfast in the misguided hope that it would offset all his many daily indulgences, in particular ice cream. Sadly, he developed heart failure and passed away at the age of 74.

Naturally, when Dad himself was diagnosed with type 2 diabetes in his fifties he was shocked; but when he managed to reverse that diagnosis by losing 9kg with his now famous 5:2 diet, it was a great relief. Over the 12 years that followed, he and my mum worked together to follow the emerging evidence as the science of weight loss evolved. The books, recipes and the programme now known as The Fast 800 are widely used around the world.

Of course, Dad was closely following the new generation of injectable weight loss drugs that had started to appear over the horizon. He was fascinated by the way the jabs were beginning to take over the diet scene, but he had significant reservations. He would have been extremely wary of the way they are being used at the moment and, had his life not been cut short, I'm pretty sure he would have been writing this book himself.

Like Dad and my mum, Clare Bailey Mosley, I am medically trained. I have long been fascinated by lifestyle medicine and for many years my focus has been on treating obesity – there's no doubt some of my parents' passion for the area has rubbed off on me.

While studying medicine at Newcastle University, I was fortunate to complete a Master of Research with Professor Roy Taylor, who was a hero of my dad's for his pioneering work with type 2 diabetes. Remarkably, Professor Taylor was able to show that type 2 diabetes, a condition that was previously thought to be a chronic and irreversible illness, could be put into remission by following a low-calorie diet. For my dissertation, I interviewed the patients who had been involved in Professor Taylor's seminal research, exploring the reasons why some were able to keep the weight off and stay out of the diabetic range, and why others struggled.

Since then, I have spent several years working as a doctor in emergency medicine in the UK and Australia, and I now work as a GP registrar. I was working in Australia when the new generation of GLP-1 (Glucagon-Like Peptide-1) weight loss medications began to make a splash on the global stage. Studies showed that semaglutide (the generic drug name for Ozempic and Wegovy) could lead to an astonishing 15 per cent sustained body weight loss in people who were overweight and living with obesity. Results like this, without dangerous side effects, had never previously been seen in a long history of weight loss drugs.

Suddenly everyone was talking about Ozempic and Wegovy, and celebrities, social media influencers and journalists flocked to take the jabs as the word spread. Semaglutide was catapulted into the limelight and quickly became a social media sensation, racking up hundreds of millions of mentions with the #ozempic hashtags on TikTok.

The weight loss jabs looked like they would be a miraculous silver bullet in the fight against obesity. But with demand so high, large parts of the market have become a lawless free-for-all. People with worrying obesity-related illnesses are self-administering the drug, and increasing their doses to eye-watering levels, without any kind of medical or nutritional advice or support. Naturally slim people are acquiring pen syringes from black-market suppliers, and using the appetite-suppressant properties to skip meals to get themselves 'beach body ready'. Others go 'on the pen' to improve their gym-honed physiques, potentially jeopardising their health. Thousands are joining unsupervised online support groups to chat with glee about how they haven't eaten anything all day other than a few biscuits in the evening, and are looking to each other for nutritional and dosage advice.

It really has become the 'Wild West' out there, with plenty of gun-slinging cowboys selling dangerous or counterfeit products for a quick profit. Although the majority of reputable online pharmacies are selling the correct product – whether that's semaglutide (Ozempic or Wegovy) or tirzepatide (Mounjaro) – their incentive seems clear: to sell as much of the product as possible and to encourage users to increase their purchase to the highest doses tolerable.

These are serious medications and, at the time of writing, we have no long-term studies to show how safe they are to take at higher doses for any protracted period of time. I'm neither for nor against these medications, but as a doctor I will always urge caution, and I will always back the science.

These jabs have arrived on the scene just in the nick of time, though. Obesity levels worldwide are completely out of control, and we have a major public health issue on our hands. In parts of Australia, they practice 'prescribed burning', which means setting controlled fires to reduce the flammable bush and grass in a bid to reduce rampant fast-moving fires later in the dry season. The focus is on acting early to prevent future disaster. Perhaps this is what the jabs will do.

For many forms of addiction or overconsumption, there are medical treatments to reduce use and so minimise long-term health problems, such as nicotine patches for smoking, and methadone for opiate addiction. These weight loss jabs could provide one powerful preventative solution to reduce the numbers of people living with obesity before obesity-related illnesses become an uncontrolled inferno.

The powerful effect of the GLP-1s on reducing appetite has highlighted for many an aspect of their internal monologue they always knew they had, but had rarely acknowledged before – 'food noise'. Food noise is the voice in your head telling you to look for your next meal or snack. It is the craving that tells you to eat that chocolate bar, even when you know you shouldn't.

It is a phenomenon that has been brought to prominence by the weight loss drugs – which appear to 'silence' them so effectively.

I share my dad's view that these jabs are likely to be an effective hammer in the toolbox to combat obesity and obesity-related illnesses. We have never had a pharmaceutical tool in the weight loss management toolbox quite like it. Some of the newest jabs on trial are so powerful, they look more like a sledgehammer!

To continue the metaphor, if you're doing a bit of DIY, a hammer is a useful tool, but it is not the only tool you need or should use. It is clear to me that these drugs are best taken to complement positive diet and lifestyle changes. Sadly, that is rarely the case at the moment. The lack of support for people taking the drugs and the shocking scarcity of advice about what to eat to ensure you get the most out of your minimised food intake is the reason I was so keen to write this book.

While the new weight loss drugs may be an excellent way to help prevent the tidal wave of obesity-related health conditions that doctors fear are heading our way, I have concerns that widespread and unsupervised use of these jabs could create a whole new set of societal health problems. Entire populations may inadvertently switch obesity for a state where they are malnourished and frail.

Our junk-food lifestyles mean we have become paradoxically overfed yet undernourished. Yes, the jabs address the fact that we are overfed, but my worry is that they may leave us even more undernourished. When you lose weight fast, you inevitably lose muscle as well as fat. Unless the millions of people taking these jabs improve the nutritional composition of their diet and take concerted care to protect and build muscle, there could be long-term repercussions for their metabolism and mobility.

The first part of this book unpicks the sinister factors that have contributed to the obesity epidemic and highlights some of the potential downstream consequences of the weight loss drugs. The second part tells you everything you need to know about this fascinating new generation of so-called miracle weight loss drugs: where they came from, how they work, their side effects and shortcomings, as well as surprising, non-weight-related benefits. Finally, in the third part I will set out how to use these medications safely and effectively to lose weight – if that's your chosen path – and keep the weight off. I unpick the latest research and speak to some of the leading experts in weight loss management, diabetes and nutrition, and look at how to eat healthy, nutritious food, while maintaining your muscle mass. It will show you how to follow a nutritious diet and healthy lifestyle to ensure the best possible long-term weight loss results.

At the back of the book, you'll find 50 easy-to-follow recipes that have been created by my mum, Dr Clare Bailey Mosley, working with the brilliant food writer Kathryn Bruton. The recipes are both delicious and easy to make, as well as packed with beneficial nutrients. You'll also find a week's worth of meal plans, to help you keep on track and get all the nutrients you need.

Whether you or someone you know is keen to try weight loss jabs, I urge you to read this book first.

# PART 1

# THE PROBLEM

It is rare for a drug to have such a large impact so quickly – to be such a focus of discussion and make so many headlines across the world. It is even more unusual for a new drug to appear to hold the answer to not just one medical issue, but many.

To understand whether these jabs really are 'miracle drugs', we need to look closely at how we got to this crisis point, and why we might be in the position even to need a miracle drug like this at all.

The problem the weight loss jabs are trying to solve is vast. The worldwide rise in obesity has created the biggest health crisis of this generation. Just like the weight gain many begin to experience as they approach middle age, the 'obesity crisis' has crept up on society insidiously. Thanks to our calorie-dense but nutritionally compromised, highly processed diets, we are experiencing a modern kind of malnutrition. One of my biggest worries is that throwing these highly powerful weight loss drugs into the mix could rapidly worsen the malnutrition issue. When or if you lose significant amounts of weight using the weight loss jabs, you could be losing a lot of muscle as well as fat, and if you go on to regain some of your lost weight, those extra pounds are more likely to be fat than muscle.

# CHAPTER 1
# THE RISE OF OBESITY

I was very skinny as an adolescent. I inherited my mum's slender frame and considered myself one of those lucky few who, no matter what they ate, couldn't possibly gain weight (though I would have preferred a bit more muscle!). But, like everyone else, I find it hard to resist sweet, salty, fatty foods and, in my first year as a junior doctor, I put on 15kg of fat, hitting 100kg in a surprisingly short timeframe. I remember one family member commenting on how impressively I had managed to 'beat the skinny gene'.

Life as a junior doctor is exceptionally busy and stressful, and I was easily tempted by strategically placed vending machines and the enticing boxes of chocolates on every ward, gifted by grateful and generous patients. Hospital canteens are not known for their nutritional output, and most of my lunches were beige. I'd while away the hour-long drive to and from work by munching on sweets and would happily scythe through a party-size bag of Doritos to myself, with a salsa dip, in front of the TV at night.

Having never had a filling in my teeth, within a year of working as a junior doctor, I'd had two. Fortunately, my fiancé is a dentist. Unfortunately, this put strain on our relationship, as it turns out she would describe me, in less polite terms, as a 'difficult' patient!

As I became more comfortable with my position in the hospital, the stress levels dropped and I was able to shift the excess weight and return to my usual baseline. I started eating well again and felt much better for it. This was helped by the fact that I was fortunate enough to have parents who taught me so much about cooking and the importance of real food. But this did show me how incredibly easy it can be to gain weight steadily in a world where you are surrounded by junk food and snacks.

## HOW WE GOT HERE

We have been watching the tidal wave of obesity creeping towards us for decades, seemingly unable to do much about it. Now, it has created the biggest health crisis of our generation. Global obesity rates have more than quadrupled since the 1990s. The numbers are simply staggering.[1] Back in the 1960s only 1 per cent of men and 2 per cent of women in the UK were living with obesity. Today, in 2024, it is 26 per cent of UK adults.[2] Across the pond in the USA, rates are even higher and have skyrocketed to 40 per cent of adults.[3] And the problem is escalating.

Carrying too much weight can significantly increase your risk of a range of diseases, such as type 2 diabetes, cardiovascular disease, high blood pressure, non-alcoholic fatty liver disease (NAFLD), certain cancers, as well as reproductive issues, osteoarthritis and more.[4] One reason for this is that obesity and an unhealthy diet can raise levels of inflammation in the body, which damages tissues and increases your risk of disease.[5] This was highlighted during the Covid-19 pandemic, when people living with obesity were found to be at an increased risk of more severe disease. I was working as a doctor in an intensive care unit at the start of the pandemic, and it was clear that the majority of those who were on ventilators with Covid complications had at least one weight-related disease. The patients in their twenties and thirties needing ventilator support were almost exclusively those with severe obesity.

Living with obesity can increase your risk of at least 13 different cancers, probably because it causes a rise in growth hormones and inflammatory signalling. It also increases circulation of hormones such as oestrogen, which can raise the risk of breast, ovarian or endometrial cancer.[6]

The risk of developing type 2 diabetes increases incrementally with weight, and in the UK 90 per cent of people with type 2 diabetes are overweight or obese. As well as increasing the chance of cardiovascular disease, diabetes is a leading cause of blindness, amputation and kidney failure. It is also associated with conditions such as depression and dementia, which is sometimes referred to by medics as type 3 diabetes.[7]

Latest estimates have found that the total cost to the UK economy of unhealthy eating, including its impact on our productivity, is a staggering £268 billion per year. This figure includes the costs of medical care, social care and the loss of productivity in people who, due to obesity and related diseases, have become too unwell to work. This cost estimate is significantly more than the entire UK National Health Service budget. Despite various attempts by governments to improve our diets, the levels of obesity have risen unrelentingly over the last few decades.[8]

Thanks to advances in modern medicine, we are living longer than ever before, though. In 1960, the average person worldwide would expect to live 54 years, today it is 73 years.[9] Good news? Perhaps not, if your latter years are dogged by ill health.

A McKinsey report estimates that half of our life is now spent in 'less-than-good health', the same proportion as back in 1960. Not surprisingly, having a substantial health problem has been found to reduce life satisfaction twice as much as other major life events, including the death of a partner or getting divorced. Sadly, our poor diet and lifestyle is playing an ever-greater role in reducing the 'healthy' and happy years of life.[10]

## IT'S NOT YOUR FAULT

Obesity has frequently been portrayed as a behavioural problem – a lack of self-control, ignorance about how to eat properly, or laziness. But, rest assured, we have not all suddenly and collectively lost willpower and become couch potatoes. Something more sinister has been going on.

Our food environment has drastically changed![11]

The Swinging Sixties were a time of huge change in the UK. They marked a period of fashion, sexual, musical and civil rights revolution and as The Beatles began to take off, so did the 'Big Food' juggernaut. This would go on to shape the next 60-plus years of our food landscape.

In search of big sales and big profits, the food industry began processing food in clever ways to entice us to buy and eat more (and more and more). As a result, today we are completely surrounded by clever concoctions of salt, fat, sugar and refined carbs that you would not see in 'whole foods' or in nature. Throw in the extra flavourings and additives, and these combinations become irresistible. They regularly activate the reward centres in our brain in a way our ancestors would not have encountered – the same reward pathways stimulated by drugs or alcohol.

This perfect combination of flavours and tastes is what's now known as the 'bliss point'. The so-called 'bliss point' is part of what encourages our overeating of processed junk foods. The worst offenders of the highly processed junk foods include those manufactured with the famous 2:1 ratio of carbohydrates to fats – the same ratio seen in breast milk.[12] These include pizza, chocolate, crisps, ice cream and cookies. These junk foods are often high in fats, sugars and salts, yet low in protein and fibre. Hyperpalatable (highly moreish!), energy dense and highly accessible, these processed foods encourage what is known as 'hedonic eating', which makes it very hard to stop. Some of these foods appear to overwhelm our appetite and portion control. As they are often low in fibre, protein and water, they are particularly edible and often fail to fill us up, or leave us hungry again shortly after eating.

But 'Big Food' had other tricks up its sleeve. It designed foods to have texture, feel, softness and even certain sounds and sights to make us eat more. The crunch of a crisp or the click of a can – many of the processed junk foods provide us with a sensory overload that we are unable to resist.

'Betcha can't eat just one' is a catchphrase synonymous with Lays crisps. It is a challenge to our willpower, knowing full well that once you've started eating a bag of their crisps, it is difficult to resist finishing it. This slogan was created back in 1963 and has lasted more than 60 years. Pringles released their own catchy version in 1991: 'Once you pop, you can't stop.' As anyone who's dug into a tube of Pringles knows, they aren't wrong. This iconic slogan highlights just how addictive these foods are. Stopping is difficult. We just want more.

We are living in a toxic 'obesogenic environment' that is playing with the reward centres in our brain and making it very difficult to eat healthily, and stop eating when we've had enough. Although our food systems have changed dramatically, our primitive, stone-age brains have not – we have, more or less, the same brains as our ancestors, but we live in a completely different food environment.

We have seen an explosion in the mass manufacturing of cheap, highly calorific, highly palatable foods. One positive outcome is that famine and starvation have become lesser issues, other than for the poorest worldwide. The average household also spends significantly less of their budget, as a proportion of their spend, on food than they did 70 years ago. However, the trade-off for all this cheap, convenient, addictive foods is rising obesity levels.

## Big plates

As our waist lines have expanded, so has the size of our dinner plates. Plates have increased from an average of 22cm to 28cm over the last 50 years. Inevitably, this means we are able to fill our plates with far more food.[13]

## SNACK ATTACK

Snacking was unheard of back in the 1960s, but it is now the norm – and you can blame 'Big Food' for encouraging that new habit too. Aggressive marketing and food shops on every street corner mean we are constantly grazing on food, something that would not have been considered normal practice 70 years ago.

According to the latest reports, the percentage of people snacking at least twice in a day has almost tripled from 27 per cent in 1977 to an astonishing 78 per cent in 2020. Snacks now account for a quarter of our energy intake and a staggering 43 per cent of our sugar intake. These days you are practically considered odd if you don't reach for a snack![14]

The problem is that the nation's favourite snacks are often loaded with refined carbohydrates, sugar, fats and salts. These soft or crunchy, fatty and salty, easily consumed snacks are often designed to bypass our feelings of fullness and can easily lead to bingeing or overeating.

Many of us are energy and time poor, so the convenience of processed junk foods often feels like a godsend. We have complicated, time-pressured lives and snacks are extremely convenient, easy to store and, most importantly, light up the pleasure centres in our brains. It is no wonder their appeal is ever rising.

The food environment has evolved in such a way as to encourage us to be passive consumers of vast quantities of delicious, moreish food. Fast-food outlets have grown exponentially across the world. Snacky junk foods have infiltrated every corner of the globe. They tick so many boxes of what we want in food – cheap, convenient, accessible, tasty and moreish. Just as it is difficult for cigarette smokers to kick the habit, many of us just can't stop eating. However, while these snacks are high in calories, they are often woefully low in nutrition, leaving us overfed but undernourished.

## WE HAVEN'T EVOLVED TO EAT LIKE THIS

Our bodies were designed to store fat to use as fuel, in order to survive during periods of famine, so we are evolutionarily wired to seek out energy-dense food. Putting on fat and eating sweet, fatty, energy-rich foods would have been beneficial during tougher times of famine. Hundreds of thousands of years ago, the ancestors who were most likely to survive would have been the ones who were most adept at doing so.

While our genes have not changed substantially over the last few millennia, the way we eat has changed dramatically. We are adapted for the savannah and the Stone Age lifestyle, not for our western diet. There is a clear mismatch, and we live in a food environment to which we are not suited. Obesity is a clear sign that our hunter-gatherer bodies are struggling.

We know there is a strong genetic element to weight and appetite. Although we clearly live in a food environment that encourages overeating, certain people are more susceptible than others. Some people may progressively gain weight when eating as little as 1,600 calories a day, when others may stay slim on 3,000 calories per day.

## Take the string test

You might think that the fatter you are, the greater your risk of type 2 diabetes, but that's not necessarily the case. It appears that we each have our own 'personal fat threshold' – once breached, negative metabolic consequences start to occur.[15]

For some, this threshold might be a relatively healthy body mass index (BMI) of 28; for others, it might not happen until they're very obese with a BMI closer to 38. At your personal threshold point, fat will start to accumulate at a greater pace around vital organs, including the liver and pancreas, leading to type 2 diabetes.[16]

The problem is 'visceral fat'. This is the excess fat that winds around your internal organs as belly fat, or around the neck, and is associated with a vast range of diseases, from type 2 diabetes to multiple cancers. It is also linked to a rise in general inflammation in the body.[17]

Think of the 'personal fat threshold' as a reservoir and dam. A dam may prevent flooding, but after a period of prolonged rainfall it, too, has its breaking point. Unfortunately, some us have a shallow reservoir and low dam. These people do not necessarily have a high BMI before fat starts 'overflowing' into the rest of the body. Others may be 'metabolically healthy' up to a BMI of 40 before their body reaches a point where the fat starts to accumulate in places we don't want it to, such as the liver. Other factors, such as age, stress and quality of diet, can also influence visceral fat accumulation.

You can accurately measure your visceral fat with a DEXA (dual-energy X-ray absorptiometry) scan, but one do-it-yourself test called the 'string test' will give you a surprisingly good estimate.

Cut a piece of string so it is as long as you are tall. Then fold the string in half and try to wrap it around your middle. In an ideal world your waist size should be less than half of your height but, if you struggle to make the ends meet, then it is likely you are carrying too much abdominal or visceral fat.

## A LITTLE WEIGHT LOSS GOES A LONG WAY

You might think you need to lose loads of weight to see improvements in your health, but the very good news is that, according to studies of obese patients, any weight loss greater than five per cent of your body weight can significantly improve your quality of life by reducing underlying health conditions. Five per cent weight loss is equivalent to a person weighing 100kg losing 5kg. Those 5kg are enough to reduce your risk of type 2 diabetes, blood pressure, lipid levels, risk of getting cancer and improve sleep.[18]

If you are living with obesity, 10 per cent weight loss is better still. One study showed that an 11 per cent loss in body weight resulted in a 52 per cent reduction of fat in the liver.[19]

In an ideal world, the fight against the rise of obesity and its related diseases would start at government level, with regulation, improved education and the subsidising of whole foods, selected on the principles of a healthy Mediterranean-style diet. Until that happens, we have to make do with the food environment we live in and do what we can.

## Summary

- We are seeing a dramatic and alarming rise in obesity worldwide, caused by a food environment that encourages overeating and continual snacking.
- Processed junk foods (with their perfect combination of sugar, carbs, fats and flavourings) have been designed to encourage

over-consumption. If you find it difficult to put down that chocolate bar or stop eating that family-sized bag of crisps, you are not alone!

- Obesity causes serious, life-limiting health problems but, for those living with obesity, losing just 5 per cent of your total body weight should lead to a reduction in heart attacks, strokes, type 2 diabetes, cancer, NAFLD and obstructive sleep apnoea.

# CHAPTER 2

# A PARADOX – OVERFED YET UNDERNOURISHED

There is growing concern that one of the main reasons so many people are putting on weight is because they are relying heavily on cheap, highly processed food, which is packed with sugar, refined carbs and fat.

Being overweight is bad enough for your health, but doctors are now observing that people who rely heavily on processed food are very often overweight *and* nutritionally deficient. It is well known that those living with obesity are already at high risk of malnutrition. In fact, malnutrition in obesity has become so common that doctors have even coined a name for it: 'malnubesity'.

Studies show 50 per cent of people with obesity have a nutritional deficiency, most commonly micronutrient deficiencies of vitamin A, B1 (thiamine), folate (B9), vitamin D, iron, calcium and magnesium. Many will also have diets that are deficient in protein, fibre, healthy fats (like omega-3) and important phytonutrients from plants such as polyphenols.[1]

As we get into older age, the consequences of malnutrition in obesity get worse. A recent study looked at adults with an average age of 77. Of those who were obese, a third were considered actively 'undernourished'. Those who were undernourished were far less mobile, less able to care for themselves, more likely to fall and have balance issues, and more likely to be depressed.[2]

We are seeing an alarming increase in Dickensian diseases, including the childhood disease rickets (as suffered by Tiny Tim in *A Christmas Carol*). Rickets is normally caused by a lack of vitamin D, which we can get from sunlight and diet, but it can also be caused by low calcium or phosphorous. Foods such as milk or flour are fortified with vitamin D in Australia, Canada and the USA, but not in the UK. It is a disease we hoped had been banished to the Victorian era.

Doctors in Australia were baffled recently by a man who arrived at hospital with an unusual rash. The man had recently had a gastric bypass operation and was eating very little food – most of it ultra-processed. It turns out he had scurvy – the disease of sailors, explorers and pirates from the sixteenth to eighteenth centuries, which is caused by low levels of vitamin C. The reason ship-faring individuals got the disease was because of a lack of access to fresh fruit and vegetables while they were away at sea for many months at a time. Ship owners and governments would expect half of the crew to perish from this disease on a voyage.[3] In our modern era, scurvy is a rare condition, so would have been extremely low on the list of differential diagnoses for those Australian doctors.[4] And yet, we are seeing a resurgence of it today. In the UK, 171 people were admitted to hospital with the condition last year (2023). In 2011, after collapsing, an 8-year-old child died of scurvy in Wales. This is a particularly sad case, when you consider that 300 years ago military surgeon James Lind discovered it could be prevented by eating citrus fruits and that within as little as 24 hours of treatment, it is possible to see a dramatic improvement.[5]

Examples like scurvy are clearly at the extreme end of malnutrition, but vitamins and minerals play a vitally important role in our general health. For instance, we need calcium, phosphorous and magnesium to build strong bones and teeth. We need vitamins A, C and E, as well as the minerals iron, zinc and magnesium for our immune systems. Vitamin B12 and folic acid are vital for healthy red blood cell production. Iodine is required for the production of thyroid hormone, as well as being crucial for brain development. There is a long list of important functions these minerals and vitamins perform.

The downstream consequences of vitamin and mineral deficiencies are a general feeling of malaise, tiredness or brain fog. But the impacts of more severe deficiencies can range from unsteadiness on your feet, to confusion and even limb paralysis, or heart failure.

In the developed world, the most common cause of irreversible visual loss in the elderly is a condition called age-related macular degeneration (AMD), which is now known to be three times more likely to occur in people who eat a 'Western diet' of processed fried foods and refined carbohydrates. This is likely due to the damaging pro-inflammatory effect of such a diet, but it is also because, without eating fruit and vegetables, you are missing out on their antioxidant effects.[6]

---

## We're getting shorter

The 1800s, despite being an era of great economic and scientific progress, saw many people in the UK have a decline in the quality of their diet. As hundreds of thousands of people left the countryside

---

for work in the city factories, they lived in cramped, unsanitary conditions with little access to good-quality, fresh food and vegetables. The diet of workers was poor.

Since then, the average man's height in the UK (unfortunately there is too little historical data for women) has increased by a colossal 11cm, thanks to the greater availability of food, fewer childhood diseases and higher wages.[7]

However, thanks to our ever-worsening diets, the UK has slipped down the world rankings of child heights once again. A report from The Food Foundation found that the height of five-year-olds has been dropping since 2013. At the same time, obesity has increased in childhood, and type 2 diabetes has tripled in young people. By the time a child leaves primary school, one third of its year group are overweight or obese.[8]

These days, the average height of a British five-year-old boy is 112.5cm and a girl is 111.7cm. However, across the channel in France, where less fast food is consumed, the average five-year-old boy stands at a relatively towering 119.6cm and a girl at 118.4cm. At the same time, one in four five-year-old children in the UK are overweight or obese.[9]

## MODERN MALNOURISHMENT

*The Times* reports that, since 2007–8, the number of people being admitted to hospital with malnutrition have quadrupled in the UK.[10]

One reason for these nutritional deficiencies is the fact that being overweight or obese puts a strain on the body, which increases levels of harmful inflammation, and the chemical reactions that the inflammatory process triggers can lead to poor absorption and storage of micronutrients, such as the mineral magnesium. Diets high in sugar are known to deplete the body's resources of vitamins such as thiamine, too.

But the biggest factor driving malnubesity is our nutritionally poor but calorie-dense Western diet. Far too many people are getting fat because they are eating more calories than their body can process. And, because they are filling up on junk food, they are not getting the nutrients their bodies need. This means malnutrition no longer looks like the skinny wraiths of Victorian fiction; these days, it is more likely to be the child who is carrying too much weight.

The problem is, many of us are increasingly eating foods that are high in calories, yet low in protein, fibre, essential fats, vitamins, phytonutrients (more on this later) and minerals. Massive worldwide studies show processed diets are associated with higher consumption of sugar and fats, but lower consumption of protein and fibre. They are also associated with a lower intake of potassium, zinc and magnesium, as well as vitamins A, B12, C, D, E and niacin (vitamin B3).[11]

Magnesium deficiency, for instance, is strongly associated with not just poor metabolic health and obesity, but also with chronic low-grade smouldering inflammation that can cause much damage to your physical health over the long term. Magnesium deficiency is also associated with higher rates of depression and cardiovascular disease. It is a reasonable marker for a healthy diet, as foods deficient in magnesium are often processed junk foods, whereas whole nutritious foods regularly contain higher levels of magnesium.[12]

## THE PROBLEMS WITH EATING LESS JUNK FOOD

Although junk food is low in nutritional content, if you eat enough, you may just about get enough vitamins and minerals (collectively known as micronutrients) to prevent diseases of severe malnutrition, such as scurvy. However, when you start on weight loss jabs you may not even reach that very low bar. My fear is that unless we change our diets, the new jabs may exacerbate malnutrition.[13]

I spoke to a mental health worker called Adele, who used Mounjaro to lose weight. She told me about her diet: 'Obviously I'm not doing it in the healthiest way – I'm just not eating at all now. So that's not good. But I'm just not hungry. Sometimes I just won't eat the whole day.'

This is a worrying trend.

After bariatric surgery where the stomach size is dramatically reduced and appetite drops, some people have found it difficult to get sufficient protein into their diet and this can lead to not only muscle loss and frailty, but a weakened immune system, brittle nails and hair loss. Other people end up deficient in crucial micronutrients, including iron, folate, vitamin A and B12. Those who do not eat a balanced nutritious diet are clearly at far greater risk. And it is likely to be the same for the weight loss jabs.

But there's a difference. After a bariatric procedure, you are given regular blood tests to check on your nutritional intake; people who take the jabs are often left to fend for themselves.[14] When people reach for an online, unregulated and unsupervised prescription for a weight loss jab, they typically halve or even quarter their consumption of food. This very often means they eat the same low-quality, ultra-processed junk food, but in considerably smaller quantities. They might lose weight, but they will be putting themselves at serious risk of malnutrition.

Most of us are already missing out on crucial brain and body healthy nutrients, such as essential fats, proteins and fibres, vitamins and minerals, but if we eat less food and don't change what eat, this is only going to get worse.

We need to be careful – weight loss drugs may address the 'overfed' aspect of our Western diet, but they may also accelerate our 'undernourishment'.

## Summary

- The ever-growing popularity of calorie-dense but nutritionally deficient processed food means that many people are eating too many calories, becoming obese, but suffering from nutritional deficiencies.
- This has resulted in a rapid rise in malnutrition, including the return of Victorian diseases of malnutrition, such as rickets and scurvy.
- There are growing concerns that people taking weight loss jabs without nutritional advice and support will continue to eat highly processed food but in smaller quantities, thereby exacerbating their nutritional deficiencies.

# CHAPTER 3
# MUSCLE LOSS

As part of my medical training, I had to accompany a district nurse on a home visit to a man in his early sixties who was suffering from severe lung disease. On the way into his flat I saw an elderly lady storming out of her front door with her Zimmer frame, travelling at a phenomenal pace. The district nurse told me that Ethel was 102 years old, but went off for a brisk walk on her own every day. I was amazed by this woman's energy and habits. She was almost 40 years older than her neighbour, but whether through luck or her healthy habits, she was thriving.

This was a clear case of 'use it or lose it' in action!

As we grow older, our body composition changes. We tend to put on more fat, while losing muscle and bone density. The natural process of losing muscle mass as we age is known as 'sarcopenia', which derives from the Greek, meaning 'flesh poverty'. If we don't step in to work those muscles, sarcopenia can lead to poor balance, fatigue and difficulty walking, standing or even sitting up in a chair. Ultimately, sarcopenia can lead to the kind of frailty that reduces your independence and increases your risk of falls, which in an older, frail person can be fatal.

The harsh truth is that most of us reach peak muscle mass between the ages of 30 and 35, and then things start to decline gradually throughout your forties. At 50, the ageing process really kicks in and you are likely to see a more rapid decline in lean muscle and strength. By the age of 60, your decline in muscle mass accelerates yet further, to more than 10 per cent loss per decade.[1]

You can blame a combination of hormonal changes, a lack of physical activity (we tend to become more sedentary with age) and the normal process of ageing. But unless we stay active and incorporate resistance exercises (see below), this muscle wastage process is somewhat inevitable.

## MUSCLE POWER

Muscular strength is obviously very important if you are a rugby player, a heavyweight boxer or a bodybuilder. But muscle is also crucial for optimal health and vitality, too. You don't have to look like Arnold Schwarznegger, Daniel Craig or a *Baywatch* cast member to have a level of body muscle mass that confers significant health benefits, though.

Not only is muscle important in 'healthy ageing' (by helping reduce risk of frailty), it also supports our immune function, increases our basal metabolic rate (our ability to burn through the calories in the food we eat), and is vital metabolically. We might not realise it, but as our muscles flex and stretch to help us move, they soak up glucose from the blood to fuel their action and, in so doing, they help keep our blood sugar levels steady. In fact, around 80 per cent of the glucose swimming around in our blood after a meal is taken up for use or storage in the muscles.

Good muscles can improve our 'insulin sensitivity', helping protect us against a condition called insulin resistance. This is a key feature of type 2 diabetes and is caused when cells in your body stop responding properly to the hormone insulin. When we become insulin resistant, our pancreas has to pump out more and more insulin to get the same effect. Ultimately, it will often fail to cope with the insulin demands, so your body struggles to keep blood sugars within a healthy range. The end result is type 2 diabetes.

Think of insulin resistance as someone giving a talk to a huge audience. The host is on stage all day. However, as the day goes on, there is a malfunction in the loud speaker, which is becoming increasingly muffled. The host nobly continues his talk throughout the day, but he notices the fault in the speaker, so he speaks louder and louder. However, the crowd still can't hear. Similarly, our cells become increasingly unable to 'hear' the signalling of insulin to dispose of sugar from the bloodstream.[2]

Another benefit of having good, strong muscles is that they can really help to slow down the ageing process, too. Grip strength (your ability to unscrew a jar, for instance) is often used by researchers as an indicator of muscle strength throughout the body, and has been highlighted as a biomarker of ageing. Poor grip strength has been used to identify older people who are at risk of ill health. Having strong hands is associated with not just longevity, but better overall health and quality of life in older age.[34] As a result of the strong association between grip strength and overall muscle strength, it is often used in studies as a predictor of falls[5] – a major cause of injury, disability and death in older people.

## THE WORRY WITH WEIGHT LOSS JABS

One big concern is that studies show people on weight loss jabs can lose a lot of muscle. For most people who lose a significant amount of weight, whether that's on a very low-calorie diet or after bariatric surgery, on average

70–80 per cent of that weight will be fat, but 20–30 per cent of the weight lost will be lean body mass.[6] That is, unless concerted efforts are made to protect and build muscle (more on this later).

Loss of lean body mass (also known as fat-free mass) encompasses all tissue loss as you shrink down in size that isn't fat. This can include loss in blood volume, water, bone tissue or tissue from your organs. However, the main component of lean body mass loss is muscle, especially when efforts are not made to preserve it. This is why 'lean body mass loss' is often used as a proxy for muscle mass loss.

There are several reasons why this happens. In order to lose weight rapidly, you have to be consuming significantly fewer calories than your body is burning. This puts you into what is called a calorie deficit, which sets your body off in search of alternative fuel sources. These reserve tanks of energy are in the form of glycogen and fat. Glycogen is stored primarily in the liver, but you'll also find it in muscles, and this is where your body will go first, in the early days of any calorie-deficit diet. It will also target fat reserves, whittling away at your waist or your double chin.

Muscles are not usually considered to be an energy source but, when food is scarce, they can be broken down into amino acids (the building blocks of proteins), which can be burnt up and used as energy. If there is insufficient protein in your diet, the body will break down muscle tissue to use this to build and repair tissues involved in vital bodily functions – a job usually done by protein. Unlike fat and carbs, protein cannot be stored, so you need to get it from every meal. This is why eating plenty of protein is so important to help protect your muscles.

A big trial (the STEP 1 trial) of people on semaglutide (Wegovy), which was funded by the Danish pharma giant, Novo Nordisk, to showcase the impressive weight loss figures, found that after 68 weeks on the jabs, the participants had lost an average of 17.3kg. However, scans showed that, on average, 40 per cent of that lost weight was lean body mass.[7] One year later, they followed up with more than 300 of the original participants of the STEP 1 trial. What they found was that participants had gained two-thirds of the weight they had originally lost while on the drugs.[8]

In the SURMOUNT-1 trial (funded by US pharma company Eli Lilly), after participants were given tirzepatide (Zepbound/Mounjaro), lean body mass made up 25 per cent of the weight lost. This is more in line with the proportion you might experience through diet or bariatric surgery.

In both studies, the participants had regular counselling on lifestyle changes delivered by health professionals. This included encouraging a calorie deficit of 500 calories and exercise of 150 minutes per week. However, the studies did not fully clarify details about the types of food (such as protein intake) or the specific forms of exercise participants engaged in. In my opinion, unless we have identical trials, we cannot truly say which course is preferential for muscle retention.

One thing we do know is that, unless efforts are taken to preserve muscle, you could see significant muscle loss while taking these GLP-1 drugs. I spoke to Dr David Unwin, GP and Royal College of General Practitioners clinical expert in diabetes, who highlighted the problem regarding muscle loss:

'We're eating junk. And junk food tends to have less protein. So, if you're just eating junk and then eating less of it, it's likely you won't be getting enough protein. And that could lead to the loss of muscle mass.'

## No muscles? There's a drug for that

The concerns about the impact of weight loss drugs on muscle loss are so significant that even the drugs companies themselves are looking for solutions – inevitably, in the form of more drugs. US pharma giant Eli Lilly, which produces tirzepatide (Mounjaro), is currently investigating medications to help you lose fat while at the same time preserving your muscles.

Lilly is also working on a drug that is designed to mimic a protein the body makes more of during exercise, in order to improve metabolism and muscle function.[9] It has been shown to be effective at conserving muscle loss in diabetics, but these are still in the early stages of their clinical trials and their long-term safety has not been fully established. So far, they have found mild side effects, such as muscle spasms and diarrhoea, but we won't know about the long-term effects of regular use for many years.[10]

Besides, the drug is administered by slow infusion through the vein, over at least a 30-minute period – not particularly practical, easy or enjoyable to receive.

## WEIGHT CYCLING

After any rapid weight loss diet, or a period on weight loss jabs, you may eventually return to your pre-diet weight. That much we know. But what we hadn't fully appreciated is the possibility that, as you regain that weight, it is more likely to be in the form of fat than muscle. If you repeat the diet, or go back on the jabs, you could end up losing more muscle each time and gaining more fat as the weight returns.

An interesting study published in 2011 explored weight regain in post-menopausal women, after a period of weight loss. Twenty-six per cent of the total initial weight lost was lean body mass, but when the women regained the lost weight, just 12 per cent of the weight regain was lean body mass.[11] This means that when you lose weight, unless you take steps to protect your muscles, you will lose fat and muscle, and when/if you regain the weight at a later date, unless you take steps to rebuild those muscles, you are likely to gain fat.

Another study, carried out in Leicester, looked at type 2 diabetics who had lost weight. The study's results suggest weight cycling could lead to loss of muscle mass and fat mass initially, but they found that whereas the fat returned, the muscle did not.[12] As the lead author Professor Tom Yates said:

'What was particularly interesting to us was that the individuals who lost and then regained weight went on to regain all of their fat mass, but lost 1.5kg of fat-free mass (primarily muscle). This equates to about a decade of aging. This suggests that "weight cycling" may be associated with a progressively worsening body composition which could have knock-on effects for longer-term physical health.'[13]

## An example of weight cycling

Here's a potential scenario: take an ordinary 65-year-old woman who is living with obesity. Susan is unable to get weight loss medication on the NHS so she orders a course of pre-filled pens from an online pharmacy. Most of these services provide no consultation with a doctor, nutritionist, or any healthcare professional, and offer minimal advice on how to alter your lifestyle. Susan takes the medication for four months and – hurrah – she loses 15kg.

Unbeknown to her, that impressive weight loss is likely to be 9kg of fat, which is great, but also 6kg of lean body mass loss.

Because she received no ongoing care or support, like many people, when she comes off the jabs, Susan is likely to gradually regain two-thirds of the weight she initially lost over the next year. Because she is no fan of exercise, a significant proportion of that will be fat.

She may still be 5kg lighter than she was before she started the jabs, but she could be carrying proportionally more body fat and less muscle, with potential implications for her future health.

The uncomfortable truth is that when or if you return to eating more calories than you burn (a calorie surfeit), the excess energy is much more likely to be stored as fat. Fat storage is a perfectly natural passive process that happens without any effort on our part. If you want to build muscle, you have to work those muscles and eat plenty of protein. This makes exercise – specifically strength training – an extremely important part of the weight loss jab solution.

Professor Dennis Villareal, a professor at the Baylor College of Medicine in Houston, has studied muscle and metabolism for almost 25 years, and he and his team have been investigating ways to reverse frailty, focusing on obese adults. He says:

'Folks with obesity need more muscle mass to carry their body weight. When they get older, they can't compensate by producing more muscle mass, so you get sarcopenic obesity, which is the worst of both worlds.'[14]

His team's work has shown that a combination of good nutrition, aerobic and strength exercises were the most effective solutions to maintain the ability to improve functional strength and help reverse frailty.[15]

## Summary

- Muscles play a number of important roles in the body's functions, allowing movement, but also supporting the immune system and metabolism, helping to keep blood glucose levels steady and reduce risk of type 2 diabetes.
- We all lose muscle as we get older (the process is called 'sarcopenia').

- When you lose weight fast, you lose fat *and* muscle.
- But when you regain weight after a period of dieting, you are more likely to regain fat than muscle.
- Protein in the diet and resistance exercise can help minimise muscle loss and maximise muscle gain.

PART 2

# THE WEIGHT LOSS DRUGS

In this section of the book, I will take you on a fascinating journey of discovery, showing you how the weight loss jabs were created and how they work. I have been digging deep into the research to provide a rigorous and impartial analysis of their possible health risks and potential health benefits outside of weight loss.

# CHAPTER 4
# THE JOURNEY TO DISCOVERY

Over the years, many odd and ultimately failed weight loss treatments have been tried – some weird, others wonderful and a few extremely dangerous. Science developed effective treatments for high blood pressure, for diabetes, for elevated cholesterol, even for impotence, but until recently the search for an effective weight loss treatment had not only been unsuccessful but it had left a path of destruction in its wake.

Early attempts to medicate weight loss began in the nineteenth century when arsenic pills (a toxic powder previously used in rat poison) were reportedly popular. The early 1900s saw the Tapeworm Diet, which encouraged people to swallow a tapeworm cyst and wait for the tapeworm to grow. This was clearly extremely dangerous, leading to the possibility of carrying a nine-metre-long tapeworm in your gut that could cause nutritional deficiencies, pain and diarrhoea. Pork tapeworms have since been found to cause neurological complications, meningitis and even death.

My dad, Michael, was a master of TV self-experimentation. He boldly (or foolishly!) ingested cattle tapeworms as part of research exploring if tapeworms could reduce certain allergies. Several weeks later (and before they had a chance to spread) he was able to film how the tapeworms were getting on. He had managed to grow three large tapeworms – triplets in his gut – and we had a couple of new family pets (which were added to the leech he brought home from another TV program that lived in a jar in the kitchen). They were latched onto his intestine and enjoying their new home. They didn't help him lose weight, though. By the time he said goodbye to the tapeworms, he had gained 1kg. My mother, Clare, was very sceptical of the whole ordeal, saying: 'Anyone thinking of popping parasites as a weight loss device should think twice.'

Between the 1930s and 1960s, the use of amphetamines (stimulant drugs) became popular as a weight loss drug in the USA. However, although effective at suppressing the appetite, they could lead to a catalogue of horrendous side effects, including addiction, anxiety, depression, psychosis and heart problems. Today, amphetamines are categorised as a class A drug.

While working as a doctor in the 1980s, my mum remembers seeing patients who'd had their jaws wired together so they couldn't chew and who could only drink liquids and liquidised food. She told us how some found enterprising ways around their restriction by blending burgers and Mars bars. It also wasn't a long-lasting solution: when patients had the wiring removed, their weight would come bouncing back, as expected.[1]

In the early 1990s a drug called Fen-Phen appeared as an exciting and effective new weight loss medication. The drug contained fenfluramine (which stimulates production of serotonin, a neurotransmitter that helps regulate mood and appetite) and phentermine (a stimulant similar to an amphetamine). However, by 1997 it was clear that, although patients would lose weight, Fen-Phen could also cause fatal heart and lung issues. The medication was withdrawn from the market in 1997 and led to multi-billion-dollar lawsuits by victims of this dangerous drug.[2]

The list of failed weight loss medications does not stop there. In 2006, rimonabant was approved in Europe for weight loss. It worked by blocking the endocannabinoid 'mood receptor' in the brain. Although rimonabant did lead to some weight loss, it had to be withdrawn after just two years because it was found to increase depression and suicidal thoughts significantly.[3]

Rimonabant was followed by sibutramine, known under brand names including Reductil, which was the hit diet drug of the noughties in Europe, only to be withdrawn from markets worldwide due to the fact that it increased patients' risks of heart attacks and strokes.[4]

You can still get your hands on a drug called orlistat, via prescription on the NHS, which was approved to assist weight loss in 1999. It works by reducing fat absorption. It was particularly popular some years ago when eating fat was assumed to be what made people fat (when in fact sugary, starchy and ultra-processed foods were more likely to be the culprits). It had an unfortunate side effect, though – if you ate more than a small amount of fat in your diet, you were likely to be struck by sudden, inconvenient diarrhoea. One of my mother's patients, who was a bus driver, found it almost impossible to manage at work, and it's not hard to guess why.

All in all, there is a sad graveyard strewn with weight loss medication failures over the years.

## Surgical solutions

Until very recently, various forms of surgery to shrink the size of the stomach (bariatric surgery) has been the treatment of choice for people with severe obesity or suffering from obesity-related diseases. You could choose from a smorgasbord of different procedures including:

- Adjustable gastric band – an inflatable band which is placed near the top of the stomach to reduce its capacity, leaving you feeling full more easily. The band can be adjusted to control food intake.
- Gastric bypass – the majority of the stomach is surgically stapled off, leaving a small pouch that connects directly to the small intestine. This procedure both restricts intake and reduces absorption of food (which can lead to malnutrition).
- Intragastric balloon – a non-surgical procedure to insert a balloon via a tube down your throat, which is then inflated to fill your stomach and limit your food intake.
- Sleeve gastrectomy – a surgical procedure to remove 80 per cent of your stomach to reduce its size and limit production of the hunger hormone (ghrelin) and a satiety hormone (leptin).

Bariatric surgeries have been shown to be a very effective form of durable weight loss, with studies showing that four years after a gastric bypass, patients lost 27.5 per cent of their baseline weight.

Additionally, it has been shown to reverse type 2 diabetes in 80 per cent of cases.[5]

These techniques aim to reduce the amount of food a person can consume and absorb, and can be very effective for those people who find it difficult to lose weight. However, there are clear drawbacks to this approach. There are always risks associated with any major surgical procedures, including anaesthetic risks, infection, bleeding and risk of blood clots. And, long term, when you restrict the amount of food you can eat, and unless you eat the right foods, malnutrition can be a significant concern.[6]

## THE BIRTH OF WEIGHT LOSS JABS

After years of false prophets, a new candidate began to emerge from the dust of the fallen obesity treatments. Back in the 1980s, scientists were refining research into a new drug that they hoped might be a breakthrough in the treatment of type 2 diabetes. Joel Habener of Massachusetts General Hospital (MGH) started investigating glucagon, a hormone that raises blood sugar. He was studying anglerfish because they have discrete organs for making insulin. He discovered a curious peptide (peptides are the building blocks of protein) that appeared to have a similar genetic code to glucagon. At around the same time, another American researcher, Graeme Bell, discovered the same peptide in hamsters. Identified as possessing a similar sequence (a genetic blueprint) to glucagon, it was hence called Glucagon Like Peptide-1 (GLP-1).

A group of researchers at MGH, including Joel Habener and a Canadian scientist, Daniel Drucker, found a way of making GLP-1 through a process of cloning. Meanwhile, a researcher working in the same building, called Svetlana Mojsov, independently discovered the sequence of GLP-1. The three of them would go on to collaborate on a research project that would lay the foundations for the discovery of a revolutionary new drug. They were able to prove, using rats, that GLP-1 stimulates the production of the hormone insulin in the pancreas after eating a meal. This hormone triggers a number of mechanisms that help control blood sugar levels.[7] This had the potential to be a fantastically effective treatment for type 2 diabetes, which manifests as uncontrolled blood sugar levels triggered by a condition called 'insulin resistance'.

After a meal, food is broken down in the gut and glucose is extracted and released into the bloodstream. When you are healthy, your body produces insulin to bring down blood glucose levels, by removing it from the bloodstream and storing it in cells. However, excessive weight gain can lead to insulin resistance, causing cells around the body to stop responding to insulin's demands to remove glucose from the bloodstream. More and more insulin is produced by the pancreas in an effort to clear the blood of glucose. If this goes on too long, the pancreas can no longer cope with the demand for insulin and blood sugar levels get too high.

The scientists who discovered GLP-1s could see its potential in amplifying the effects of insulin, which could prove a real breakthrough in the treatment of type 2 diabetes. However, the GLP-1 naturally produced by the human body is broken down too rapidly – within minutes – so limiting its potential pharmaceutical use.[8] A solution to this appeared in an unlikely fashion.

## MEXICAN LIZARDS

An endocrinologist from New York called Dr Joseph Eng became interested in the venom of the gila monster, a poisonous lizard found in the deserts of southwestern USA and northwest Mexico, after reading a paper that revealed the venom could cause inflammation of the organ where insulin is made: the pancreas. This lizard spends 95 per cent of its life underground due to the extreme heats of its desert habitat. It can survive for extended periods without food, while maintaining stable blood sugar levels the whole time. It only eats five to ten times a year but can gorge up to 35 per cent of its body weight in a single sitting.[9] Dr Eng realised that the venom, or something in the venom, might stimulate the pancreas to produce insulin, which would explain how gila monsters could control their blood sugar levels through huge feasts and protracted periods of famine.

In 1990, he identified the substance and called it Exendin-4. Excitingly, Exendin-4, unlike GLP-1, was not rapidly degraded by the body.[10]

Meanwhile, Canadian scientist Daniel Drucker, who had been involved in the team responsible for the initial discovery of GLP-1s, was on the lookout for ways they could be used therapeutically.[11]

After reading Joseph Eng's 1992 research paper, Drucker was intrigued and decided to pursue further research into the gila monster lizard. After trying and failing to clone lizard DNA from a freezer at the Royal Ontario Museum in Toronto, he realised he would have to go straight to the source. He contacted a professional reptile handler called Bob Murphy for assistance. (Drucker later explained: 'You can't just go to a pet store and ask for a poisonous lizard.')[12]

Murphy got in contact with Utah Zoo, explaining that the gila monster lizard could be a 'silver bullet' for the treatment of diabetes. The zoo promptly flew one lizard in a wire cage to Toronto and Exendin-4 was extracted from the lizard's saliva.

Through this exercise, Drucker was able to show that, while GLP-1 in its natural form is broken down in minutes, Exendin-4 lasts several hours before being metabolised. His work added to the body of evidence that this hormone could be used for the treatment of type 2 diabetes.[13]

Considering the significance of this discovery, it is surprising that Drucker struggled to drum up interest. In an interview in the *New York Times*, he described his pursuit as 'a pretty lonely field'.[14] Although he applied to give talks with the Endocrine Society, he was given one of the last slots of the day and spoke to an almost empty lecture hall. As he explained in an interview for Canadian magazine *Macleans*: 'There were already pills you could take to stimulate insulin secretion, so people were like, "Why would you inject something that comes from a poisonous lizard?" '[15]

In the meantime, back in New York, Dr Joseph Eng was busy trying to patent his Exendin-4 and was coming up against resistance of his own. When he discovered the hormone in 1990, he was working at the Bronx Veterans Administration Medical Center, but they declined his request for this to be patented as a drug for type 2 diabetes because they were solely focused on treating war veterans and retired military personnel, and felt any patents had to address warfare-related injuries.

So, at great personal expense, Eng resorted to hiring his own patent lawyers to approve the patent, but confessed to having problems paying the patent bills, complaining that, 'Developing a drug candidate requires hundreds of millions of dollars. I don't have the resources, or the expertise, or the access to people who do.'[16]

Just like an author who has to self-publish, or a singer–songwriter who releases their own music without the backing of a record label, Eng had to fight to establish his patent for his drug discovery. Even when he got his patent, the pharmaceutical companies showed no interest. Then, in 1996, he finally had a breakthrough and was able to licence his work to a small biopharmaceutical company called Amylin. Together they created a synthetic version of Exendin-4 called exenatide. By 2005, exenatide, under the brand name Byetta, was approved by the FDA (US Food and Drug Administration) for the treatment of type 2 diabetes.[17]

And that's when the fun really started. Over time, it was becoming evident that GLP-1 didn't just help manage blood sugar levels, but it prompted weight loss in people *without* diabetes.[18]

During this period, Novo Nordisk got FDA approval for a long-acting GLP-1 injection called liraglutide (which you had to inject daily). The numbers were impressive, but not spectacular. Then, in 2017, Novo Nordisk got a weekly jab called semaglutide (under the brand name Ozempic) approved by the FDA for blood sugar control in patients with type 2 diabetes. Very quickly, trials started to show promising weight loss effects on people *without* diabetes too.[19]

That's when the world really started talking about the possible potential of GLP-1.

Some of the most impactful drug discoveries have been made when medications intended for one use have been shown to be effective in other domains. For instance, Viagra was originally used to treat high blood pressure but became the blockbuster drug of the 1990s when it was discovered it was also extremely effective at treating erectile dysfunction.

## THE JABS HIT THE BIG TIME

The greatest leap forward happened as a result of a big study published in 2021 (the STEP 1 trial, which was funded by Novo Nordisk). It was a randomised, double-blind trial exploring the weight loss effect of a higher dose of semaglutide than had been used for type 2 diabetics. When used for type 2 diabetes, the maximum dose is 1mg, but the weight loss dose for this study was ramped up to 2.4mg. One group got the semaglutide and the other group got a placebo. Both groups were advised to eat healthily and exercise. The participants were obese or overweight, but not diabetic. After 16 months, the group on semaglutide lost an average of 15 per cent of their body weight, but the placebo group only lost 2.4 per cent. Previously, any weight loss drug that could lead to more than 5 per cent weight loss was considered a 'success', so this was a truly remarkable, unprecedented result. Although the same drug, the weight loss version (given at a higher dose) was called Wegovy. However, to this day it remains better known as 'Ozempic'.

Ozempic/Wegovy (semaglutide) exploded onto the world scene as the latest and, at the time, best weight loss drug on the market. Famous early adopters included Rebel Wilson, who credited the GLP-1s with aiding her 36kg weight loss, and Oprah Winfrey, who told TV viewers: 'You weren't thinking about the food! You weren't obsessing about it!'[20] Elon Musk credits semaglutide with his own 13.6kg weight loss, too.[21] Having utilised the GLP-1s himself, Musk has recently stated on his platform X: 'Nothing would do more to improve the health, lifespan and quality of life for Americans than making GLP inhibitors super low cost to the public.'[22]

Ozempic/Wegovy became the hot weight loss ticket sought after by many Hollywood A-listers, and it has frequently made newspaper headlines worldwide. Its popularity was so extreme that it led to global shortages for diabetic patients, many of whom had been taking semaglutide for years. The rise in Ozempic's sales, and resulting profits, was so great that, as of December 2024, Novo Nordisk is by far the largest company in Europe, worth $384 billion.[23]

Meanwhile, the American pharma giant Eli Lilly started researching the efficacy of combining GLP-1 with Glucose-Dependent Insulinotropic Polypeptide (GIP) as a 'dual agonist' on weight loss. They discovered a new drug they called tirzepatide (the brand name is Mounjaro or Zepbound), which acts in a similar way to reduce appetite, slow the digestive tract and help control blood sugar levels.

Eli Lilly's studies also showed that tirzepatide reduced the progression from pre-diabetes to type 2 diabetes by an incredible 94 per cent. Not only did participants see improving blood sugar levels, but they also saw improvements in other risk factors for heart disease and strokes, including improved blood pressure, cholesterol and reduced waist size.[24]

A study published in 2022 (the SURMOUNT-1 trial) found those given the highest dose of tirzepatide (15mg), lost an average of almost 23 per cent of their body weight over a three-year period, compared to just 2 per cent for those taking the placebo.

The level of weight loss achieved by these medications was beyond Novo Nordisk and Eli Lilly's wildest dreams. These blockbuster drugs have already enabled them to make huge profits, with more expected in the future. Reuters have forecast the market for these weight loss drugs to have reached more than $100 billion by 2030.[25]

Clinical trials are already underway for a *triple* agonist, which could lead to even higher levels of weight loss.

## FUTURE DEVELOPMENTS

It is becoming clear that these jabs are no passing fad. I'm convinced that the GLP-1s will only become a bigger, more prominent part of our lives. They will inevitably become more affordable, accessible and increasingly prevalent in society, as new and improved medications come to the market. Although earlier GLP-1 drugs did show promise in increasing weight loss, Ozempic was the first of the true heavy hitters of the weight loss drugs. However, it is far from the last, as bigger and better solutions overtake it, in terms of magnitude of weight loss. At the moment there are more than 20 drugs known to be in development, and dozens more to come.

Currently there's a lot of hype around CagriSema, a weekly jab combining semaglutide with cagrilintide (this mimics amylin, a hormone that helps you feel full after eating) and produced by the original creators of semaglutide, Novo Nordisk. Not yet being sold to the public, the expectation had been that the results would show roughly 25 per cent weight loss. When the numbers from the trial came in at 22.7 per cent body weight loss, the stock dropped in value and investors wiped $125 billion off the valuation of Novo Nordisk. With competition this hot, Wall Street can be a ruthless bunch.

When studies showed that people on tirzepatide (Mounjaro) lost more than 20 per cent of their body weight, it was dubbed the 'King Kong' of weight loss medications. But we are now looking down the line at a *triple* agonist – retatrutide.

Retatrutide is showing even higher levels, on average 24 per cent weight loss, when given at the higher dose. Yet this weight loss was achieved in less time – just 24 weeks, as reported in the *New England Journal of Medicine* last year.[26] It mimics GLP-1 and two other hormones (GIP and glucagon) – this triple hit appears to have a synergistic, amplifying effect at reducing appetite, leading to greater weight loss.

Clinical trials suggest this medication may lead to even more weight loss than Mounjaro. In fact, the studies suggest that those taking this medication lose almost as much as someone undergoing bariatric surgery. If Mounjaro is the 'King Kong' of weight loss, perhaps retatrutide will be 'Godzilla'.

What if weekly injections are too much? Well, researchers are working on a monthly jab. Biotech company Amgen are in phase 2 trials for a medication that can be given monthly. It activates the GLP-1 receptor, while blocking the GIP receptor. Trials have shown that the medication called MariTide led to 20 per cent body weight loss after one year.[27] There is also research going into an injection to be given just once every three months.[28]

Other research is progressing to produce a version of semaglutide (Ozempic) in pill form. When taken orally, semaglutide has to be consumed at around 200 times the injection dose, as less than 1 per cent of the GLP-1 agonist is absorbed by the gut. When given at this high oral dose, it appears to be as effective as it is in its injected form. For those who don't wish to be jabbed every week, this could one day provide a useful alternative solution.[29]

## Summary

- Numerous weight loss treatments have been tried over the years, including arsenic pills, tapeworms, jaw wiring, amphetamines and bariatric (stomach reducing) surgery.
- Weight loss jabs started life in the 1980s as a treatment for type 2 diabetes.
- In 2021, a study showed that larger doses of the GLP-1 injections that diabetics were using to control their blood sugar levels could cause dramatic weight loss.

# CHAPTER 5

# HOW THE WEIGHT LOSS MEDICATIONS WORK

## FOOD NOISE

The meteoric rise in popularity of weight loss jabs has brought a new phrase into the modern vocabulary – 'food noise'. This refers to the internal chatter many people experience when it comes to food and hunger. Some lucky souls rarely 'hear' it, but plenty of other people live with a near-constant, rolling, food-related dialogue in their heads: they can't stop themselves thinking about planning their next meal, imagining the taste of it, wanting to eat it, or just looking at images of food online.

On a basic level, we need food noise in order to survive – it is all part of the message signalling that goes from our gut to our brain, telling us we are hungry and must take in some fuel. But for many people, food noise is so incessant and intrusive that it drives over-eating and a very unhealthy obsession with food.

When the jabs were trialled for weight loss, the makers marvelled at how successfully they dull people's appetite, but it has only been since so many people have been using them that the full impact has been realised. For many users, the jabs either hugely reduce food noise or they silence it altogether. Then, when you do eat, some users report being more inclined to crave healthy and wholesome food – the thought of booze or anything fatty or sugary makes them feel queasy. This factor alone makes the food restriction required for rapid weight loss so much easier to tolerate. I spoke to a number of people who had taken the jabs as part of my research for this book, and many talked about the relief when they noticed their food noise had been switched off. One of them, Adele, a smiley, enthusiastic mental health worker, who lost three stone in three months after taking Mounjaro (tirzepatide), described how the persistent food noise she lived with all her life disappeared: 'You know when you're at the supermarket and you walk past the sweets at the checkout and put them in your basket? I don't do that any more. I used to think about food all the time and I just don't any more. I'd go to the shop at night after a shift and buy snacks, then go home and eat the lot. I was rarely hungry, it was just eating for the sake of eating. I don't do that any more either.'

## Has food addiction been driving food noise?

It is clear that some people hear food noise more loudly than others, but I suspect our obesogenic food environment has massively turned up the volume for many of us. Food scientists have spent years exploiting the perfect combination of refined carbohydrates, fats and flavourings to overload the reward pathways in our brains to make processed foods irresistible. These foods stimulate our hedonic hunger, they overwhelm our appetite control on purpose, so we just can't stop ourselves thinking about them.[1]

We are increasingly recognising that ultra-processed foods (UPFs) can be as addictive as cigarettes or alcohol. Multiple studies have shown that hyperpalatable foods trigger similar brain systems to those triggered by addictive drugs. Both addictive drugs and hyperpalatable foods cause a reduced responsiveness in our brain reward systems over time, meaning that we need more and more of them to get that same hit of feel-good hormones, such as dopamine. This ultimately leads to a compulsive overconsumption of that addictive substance, be it factory-produced cookies, or cocaine.[2]

In natural, minimally processed foods, you rarely see anything like the ratio of carbohydrates to fats that you see everywhere in UPFs. Crisps and chocolate contain that magic 2:1 ratio of carbohydrates to fat that sends the brain haywire. And that is before you consider all the extra additives that make ultra-processed junk foods so delicious. It's no wonder the food noise shouts so loud and cravings are sent spiralling out of control![3]

## FOOD NOISE IS LOUDER FOR SOME

While food noise is universal and can be experienced by anyone, the intensity can vary from person to person. WeightWatchers and the STOP Obesity Alliance conducted a study[4] to better understand food noise and its impact on those who have weight struggles. It showed that 57 per cent of people who were either overweight or obese experienced continued and disruptive thoughts about food.

Of those questioned, 67 per cent of obese participants said they wished they didn't think about food as often as they did, compared to 48 per cent of those who fell into a healthy weight range. Similar numbers of obese respondents said they had constantly to fight the urge to eat even when not hungry and that the food noise made it difficult to stick to a weight loss plan. By contrast, the same study revealed that when it came to obese people using weight loss jabs, 69 per cent said they no longer obsessed over their next meal or snack, while 58 per cent said they had improved focus.

For many who are overweight or living with obesity, food noise can be confounding, with 65 per cent stating they fight the urge to eat even though they aren't hungry.

James Corden opened up about his own experience with Ozempic on his Sirius XM radio show: 'I tried Ozempic for a bit, but it didn't work. It takes away your hunger, but I realised nothing about my eating habits was linked to being hungry. I am very rarely eating just because I'm hungry.'

It is clear that food noise can be a significant roadblock to weight health, with 61 per cent of people living with obesity or being overweight saying that food noise makes it difficult to stick to a nutrition or exercise plan.

During a chat on the podcast 'How to Fail', TV presenter Richard Osman spoke of his own food addiction. He described it as the 'drum beat' of his life: 'Alcoholics will tell you the same, like it's absurd that there's a bottle of vodka in front of you or there's a packet of crisps in front of you and it's more powerful than you.'[5]

An international report of 281 studies from 36 countries showed that food addiction was seen in 14 per cent of the population, the same percentage addicted to alcohol, while 18 per cent were addicted to smoking. Half of those with a binge-eating disorder fit the criteria for food addiction.[6] I have seen patients suffering with depression and anxiety, who informed me that they binge eat 'just to feel something'. For some, binge eating is about filling a void.

When he was in his forties, my dad (Michael) was a self-confessed chocolate addict. I'll never forget one Easter when I was about ten, my siblings and I ran downstairs to hunt for our chocolate eggs only to be find they had all gone. After a small amount of investigating, to our horror we discovered our father had eaten them the night before. Now if that's not addiction, I don't know what is! As he approached middle-age, Dad swapped his milk chocolate for dark chocolate, which he found far less addictive, and then, after reversing his type 2 diabetes in 2012, my parents focused on keeping most of his temptations out of the house.

## EMOTIONAL EATING

Not only are our foods addictive, but research shows that living with obesity can cause changes in the brain that affect our relationship to food. Food addiction is just as challenging as many other types of addiction. You could argue that it's even harder to manage because you can't be abstinent as you still have to eat. And to make it even more difficult, we are surrounded by temptation. In fact, UPFs now make up more than half our diet.

Recent research has shown us what we have suspected for some time, that emotional triggers can influence our eating habits. When we are stressed, we typically favour energy-dense hyperpalatable foods, particularly those high in fat and sugar.[7]

This is why during stressful periods, particularly during chronic stress, we'd rather reach for the cookies or crisps than cook a healthy meal. You can see how this could lead to a vicious cycle of consumption whereby, because we are stressed, we eat unhealthy processed foods, leading to worsening stress and further dysregulated eating.[8]

Stress can affect the signalling of satiety hormones, including GLP-1 and another called leptin.

## How the jabs work

It is fascinating that the GLP-1 weight loss jabs seem to be so effective at silencing food noise, and they appear to help reduce our cravings for hyperpalatable junk food. They act not just on our appetite but on reward processing, too. Many people have seen a huge reduction in their binge-eating behaviours while taking the jabs, because they inhibit our 'reward pathways' in the brain.

Currently, the two most popular weight loss drugs on the market are semaglutide (Ozempic) and tirzepatide (Mounjaro). Both drugs act in a similar way by reducing appetite, slowing down the digestive tract and helping to control blood sugar levels. This is how they work:

*Silencing food noise*
The body's control of eating is primarily driven by two key regulatory mechanisms: hunger-induced eating and reward-related eating. Reward-related eating, also known as 'hedonic eating', is what often drives us toward hyperpalatable junk foods. This can influence

cravings and push us to eat. Some people only experience so called 'food noise' and the drive to seek food when they are hungry. Others admit to thinking about food throughout the day, even when they are full. The volume and intensity of 'food noise' is very variable from person to person.

The weight loss drugs can reduce food noise in several ways. Firstly, by increasing feelings of fullness, which will inevitably make you less focused on food. Reducing your appetite decreases cravings and makes food thoughts less intrusive. Evidence suggests that they also adjust our food-related behaviours by activating key areas of the brain in order to reduce reward-seeking behaviours and so reduce our food consumption.[9] This helps us to regulate our motivation to seek out food, such as a bag of crisps or a chocolate bar, and consume it.

It is GLP-1's effects on the brain that have led to the important discovery that it could reduce problematic reward-seeking behaviours in addiction to substances, including alcohol and recreational drugs, and not just food. The exact mechanisms are still unclear, but it appears to affect reward pathways in the brain, influencing dopamine-driven cravings. Dopamine is a neurotransmitter (a chemical messenger) involved in reward-motivated behaviour. Research in rodents shows how activation of GLP-1 receptors regulates dopamine in reward centres of the brain, such as the nucleus accumbens. This suppresses the desire to seek out and eat palatable foods, which would cause you to be less 'food motivated' and seek less food. GLP-1s appear to reduce our response to typical food cues, for instance the sight and smell of processed junk foods.[10]

A 2024 study on mice found that while semaglutide reduced food-seeking behaviour, it enhanced dopamine signalling related to the pleasure of eating, and resulted in the consumption of less sucrose.[11]

A 2015 study in humans showed a fascinating insight into how the GLP-1s appear to modulate these reward pathways in a nuanced way. Using MRI brain scans, they found reduced activation of reward pathways in *anticipation* of a tasty treat. In the case of this 2015 study, that treat was chocolate milk. However, they found *increased* activation of these same pathways on *consumption* of that chocolate milk. What this suggests is that you are less likely to seek out hyperpalatable junk foods due to reduced cravings, but if you do consume them, you will be more easily satisfied by a smaller quantity of food, which should reduce overeating.[12, 13, 14, 15]

## Reducing appetite

There are multiple important hormones involved in leaving us feeling full, and others that make us hungry, but the GLP-1 drugs have been shown to act on the brain to reduce appetite dramatically.[16] They work by mimicking the naturally occurring versions of the gut peptides GLP-1 and GIP, which are hormones naturally secreted by the human body in response to food. While semaglutide acts on one receptor (GLP-1), tirzepatide acts on two receptors (GLP-1 and GIP). It is thought the two complement each other and work together synergistically. GLP-1 can pass through the blood–brain barrier, and acts on the brain to reduce appetite and increase satiety. It appears to stimulate key areas of the brain, such as the hypothalamus, which is responsible for the control of many hormones in the body, and acts as the body's thermostat. It also plays a key role in the regulation of body weight.[17]

### Regulating fat storage

The jabs can improve the way your body metabolises and stores fat.[18] Recent research suggests that both GLP-1 and GIP may play a role in fat metabolism in the body. These hormones appear to act on the adipose tissue (the fat cells in our body), helping to reduce the formation of new fat (lipogenesis). They also encourage fat burning by a process called 'browning', which means turning white fat tissue to brown fat tissue. This can lead to fat loss overall, because brown fat is metabolically active (it is used to create heat, which burns calories), whereas white fat just stores energy.

### Slowing digestion

After we eat a meal and it enters our stomach, one of the GLP-1/GIP's first actions is to slow the emptying of our stomach into the small intestine. This prevents rapid blood sugar spikes and also helps you feel fuller and more satisfied after eating less.

*Smoothing out blood sugar spikes*

GLP-1 binds to receptors in the pancreas to stimulate the release of the hormone insulin. Insulin then helps reduce the amount of sugar in the blood, enabling us to maintain stable blood sugars within the normal ranges.[19, 20]

GLP-1 acts as an 'amplifier' of insulin, helping our bodies to bring down blood sugar levels, directly in response to eating food. When you are living with obesity, this amplifying effect is naturally dampened down (this is called 'insulin resistance'), but the jabs act like a megaphone, revving up the process. While amplifying insulin, GLP-1s also reduce levels of a hormone called glucagon, which would normally raise blood sugar.

## Summary

- 'Food noise' is a new term coined to describe the food-related chatter that can fill people's minds.
- The proliferation of modern ultra-processed foods makes food addiction and food noise more likely.
- Food noise is louder for some people than others.
- One of the key ways the new weight loss jabs appear to work is by silencing food noise.
- The jabs also reduce appetite, regulate fat storage, slow digestion and smooth blood sugar spikes.

# CHAPTER 6

# SIDE EFFECTS AND RISKS

Even in the modern world of medicine, there is rarely such a thing as a 'free lunch'. Like most medications, the GLP-1s come with side effects. These can vary from person to person and spread from the mildly inconvenient (sulphur burps) to the deadly. Fortunately, for most people, the side effects are mild, but for some they can be severe and dangerous.

## NAUSEA AND VOMITING

The most common complaints about GLP-1s are gut-related symptoms. Early studies showed nearly half of the people (four in ten) taking the lowest 2.4mg dose of semaglutide (Ozempic) experienced nausea, and a quarter vomited.

Each person reacts differently, but if you eat too much when you're taking the jabs, the side effects can be brutal. Anecdotally, it seems that eating too much processed junk food can trigger symptoms, possibly because it is easier to stop eating real food when you feel full, whereas UPFs are designed to encourage you to keep on eating. Too much alcohol can cause problems, too.

For some, the nausea gradually goes away as your body learns to tolerate the drugs, but for others, such as actor Stephen Fry, who lost 31kg in weight, this was not the case: 'The first week or so, I was thinking, "This is astonishing. Not only do I not want to eat, I don't want any alcohol of any kind. This is going to be brilliant." '[1] But the longer he took the drug, the worse his symptoms got. Fry describes getting 'sicker and sicker' to the point where he was 'literally throwing up four, five times a day' and he eventually had to stop.

Former Prime Minister Boris Johnson has also written about his experiences with GLP-1s: 'For weeks I jabbed my stomach, and for weeks it worked. Effortlessly, I pushed aside the puddings and the second helpings. "Wasn't it amazing," I said to myself, "how little food you really need." I must have been losing four or five pounds a week – maybe more – when all at once it started to go wrong. I don't know why, exactly. Maybe it was something to do with constantly flying around the world and changing time zones, but I started to dread the injections, because they were making me feel ill. One minute I would be fine, and the next minute I would be talking to Ralph on the big white phone; and I am afraid that I decided that I couldn't go on.'[2]

## EGGY BURPS

One in ten people have reported suffering from 'Ozempic burp', which is a specific type of eggy, sulphurous-smelling burping.[3] This probably happens because the drug slows down the digestive system, leaving food to linger longer (allowing stinky bacteria to grow), or it could be that the drug itself is increasing levels of sulphur-producing bacteria in the gut. Fizzy, carbonated drinks may be best avoided, too, as they can worsen excessive burping.

## DIARRHOEA

There are GLP-1 receptors occupying the full length of the gut, so some people can experience problems at the end of the line, too.

In the same Ozempic study, just under a third of respondents reported having diarrhoea. I spoke to Tanya, a retired GP, who was prescribed tirzepatide (Mounjaro) by an online pharmacy. She says she lost weight on the starter dose (2.5mg) with no problems but was advised to increase her dose to 7.5mg after a couple of months. 'That was a really bad month or two because I had very bad side effects – catastrophic squits. And that was really off-putting. Plus, I did not feel like doing any exercise. I thought, this is stupid, I'm finding it really difficult to eat much. I'm not exercising. This is the opposite of what I think is okay on a weight loss plan.'

## CONSTIPATION

A quarter of people on the drugs are likely to experience constipation caused by the slowing of the transit of food through the gut. Eating fibre and drinking plenty of water is important to help reduce the risk of constipation. More on this later (page 144).

---

### Case study

Peter is in his mid-seventies. He is retired and previously worked in the automotive industry. He started semaglutide four years ago in an attempt to reverse his type 2 diabetes and successfully lost more than 19kg. He told me: 'I have a very sweet tooth and that's not an ideal thing for a diabetic. At first the results were terrifying! I was

---

exploding in every direction from every possible orifice – that's what happens if you 'misbehave' and continue to eat like you did before. But then I got my head around it and now I eat about a third of what I used to consume. The side effects stopped.

'I found there was a direct correlation: eat too much and you'll be ill. So now there's a bit of fear factor – I worry that if I eat too much, I will suffer for it in a dramatic and most embarrassing way, so I don't do that any more.'

## Ozempic face (and bottom)

Suddenly slim Hollywood stars have been so facially transformed, that social media has coined the term 'Ozempic face' to describe an alarmingly gaunt appearance. This can happen as fat and muscle are lost from the face, and the skin, stretched for years by rounded cheeks, starts to sag as the 'elastin fibres' (the protein in your skin that gives it its elasticity) lose their ability to 'retract' when the fat melts away.

A similar affliction is 'Ozempic butt' (a flat, dropped bottom) caused by muscle wastage and fat loss around your glutes and quads, if you don't do enough exercise to protect those important muscles.

## WEIGHT LOSS ADDICTION

Pictures of TV personality Sharon Osbourne have shown how she dropped to an extremely low weight after taking weight loss jabs. She revealed that she had lost 19kg and was struggling to control the weight loss.

'My warning is – don't give it to teenagers, it's just too easy,' she told the *Daily Mail*.[4] 'You can lose so much weight and it's easy to become addicted to that, which is very dangerous. I couldn't stop losing weight and now I can't afford to lose any more. I need to put on ten pounds but, however much I eat, I stay the same weight.'

People respond to the GLP-1s differently and it is difficult to say exactly why Sharon Osbourne has taken things further than she wanted. It could be a natural change in appetite, which many people experience as they get older, and is linked to a change in the balance of key hunger hormones (ghrelin) and satiety hormones (leptin). Having lost 19kg, it is likely she will have lost muscle, too, which could further reduce her body's demands and appetite.

Additionally, as she has admitted, it is easy to become 'addicted' to the weight loss, which can be dangerous and is a major worry for others using the drug, as it becomes more and more mainstream.

These drugs were not designed for someone like Sharon Osbourne – she would be unlikely to fit the guidelines for prescribing these drugs for weight loss (a BMI of at least 27 plus a weight-related health problem). Weight loss drugs can be more dangerous for people in the 'normal' BMI range.

## LOSS OF JOY IN FOOD

There are anecdotal reports online of people on the jabs who lose all their joy in food. If the GLP-1s sap our hedonic drive for food, they also have the potential to make food less enjoyable. Danish Professor Jens Juul Holst was an important researcher in the discovery of GLP-1s in the 1980s. He admitted in a recent interview with the magazine *Wired*: 'Once you've been on this for a year or two, life is so miserably boring that you can't stand it any longer and you have to go back to your old life.'

---

### Will the jabs affect our relationships?

Perhaps restaurant menus will change to accommodate our smaller appetites, or perhaps the sociable concept of eating together will fall away entirely. The drugs could certainly impact our desire to meet up with friends in a restaurant or at a dinner party. And the drugs might sound the death knell for wavering romantic relationships, if they follow a similar pattern to the phenomenon of 'bariatric divorce', where weight loss in one partner can lead to conflict and resentment in the other.[5]

---

## SUICIDAL THOUGHTS AND DEPRESSION

Anecdotally, people taking the medications have described feeling 'flat' and there were concerns it could increase depression. More worryingly, there have been concerns that it could cause suicidal thoughts. The concern is understandable, especially given that the weight loss medications affect our reward systems and pleasure-seeking behaviours. But the evidence seems to suggest that the *opposite* is in fact true.

The initial breakthrough STEP-1 trial, that looked at semaglutide, found a small but significant *reduction* in depression symptoms in those taking semaglutide.[6] Another study found a 49–73 per cent reduction in suicidal thoughts in those taking semaglutide, compared to other diabetic medications.[7] The improvement in symptoms of depression may be directly due to the weight loss or even the improvement in metabolic health.

It is interesting to note that there is an established bi-directional relationship between depression and obesity – which means obesity increases the risk of depression, but depression also increases the risk of obesity. Type 2 diabetes is also a major risk factor for developing depression. If you have type 2 diabetes, you have a two-fold increased likelihood of depression compared to the general population.[8]

## SERIOUS ISSUES TO WATCH OUT FOR

### Slowing the gut and blockage of the bowel

Gastroparesis is a condition sometimes referred to as 'stomach paralysis' and some studies suggest that GLP-1s can cause a 66 per cent increased risk of gastroparesis.[9] In the same way that the GLP-1s can slow stomach emptying, it can also slow the bowel to the point where it temporarily stops working and no longer allows food to pass through. This is called paralytic ileus.

In studies on mice, high doses of GLP-1s have been shown to increase the size of the bowel, leaving it increasingly inelastic and scarred, potentially increasing the risk of blockages of the bowel known as bowel obstructions.[10] Bowel obstructions like this are potentially dangerous, very painful and can be life threatening if not properly treated, as they can lead to strangulation of the bowel.[11] One real-world study of 25,000 type 2 diabetics found a three-and-a-half-fold increased risk of bowel obstruction associated with GLP-1 usage.[12]

Dr David Unwin warned me about a GLP-1 patient he had seen: 'This person ended up in intensive care because his gut had simply shut down – parts of it just stopped working. For that individual, the consequences were very serious and he was in hospital for a very long time.'

## Pancreatitis

Another disease that has been linked to the GLP-1s is acute pancreatitis. This is a particularly nasty, painful and potentially fatal condition where the pancreas, which sits below the ribs, becomes inflamed. The pain can be so severe that on a scale of one to ten, it can hit the highest pain level ten, often requiring strong pain killers, such as morphine. A British woman recently died of the condition. Susan McGowan, a nurse working for the NHS in Glasgow, had started tirzepatide. After two doses of the medication, she was admitted to hospital with acute pancreatitis and multiple organ failure. Sadly, days after being admitted, she died.[13] The 'use of prescribed tirzepatide' was highlighted as a contributing factor in Susan's death.

In clinical trials when used for the treatment of type 2 diabetes, Mounjaro (tirzepatide) was associated with a twofold increased risk of pancreatitis, when compared to other diabetes treatments. However, the risk remains low at 0.2 per cent in patients taking the jab for weight loss purposes (the same as a placebo).[14]

The evidence is mixed. One meta-analysis that looked at multiple trials found no clear association between pancreatitis and GLP-1s.[15] Other large meta-analysis studies have found no greater risk of pancreatitis from taking semaglutide, compared to a placebo.[16] In rare instances, it may be that some of the GLP-1 medications can trigger pancreatitis, but the absolute risk remains low.

Still, US and EU drug regulators currently warn that caution should be exercised with anyone with a history of pancreatitis, and if pancreatitis is suspected, the drug should be discontinued and not restarted.[17]

## Gallstones

Rapid weight loss is known to increase the risk of gallstones and this appears to be true of weight loss medication, too.[18] This is likely to be because the gall bladder releases bile and as the GLP-1s slow down the emptying of the gall bladder, it makes it more likely that the hardened material is allowed to collect and form gallstones.[19]

A large meta-analysis found an overall 27 per cent increased risk of gallstones in those taking GLP-1s, and a 56 per cent increased risk of gall bladder disease for those using GLP-1s at the higher weight loss dose (rather than at a lower dose for type 2 diabetes). This included infection, inflammation and blockage of the gall bladder. Sudden-onset severe pain in your upper abdomen (below the centre of your rib cage) or in the upper right corner could indicate gallstones and would need medical attention.

## Thyroid cancer

For the last few years, there has been considerable concern that GLP-1s may cause thyroid cancer, after a study showed a link between the GLP-1s and thyroid cancer in rats. However, the evidence in humans is inconclusive. Some meta-analyses, pooling many different studies together, have found a small increased risk of thyroid cancer. However, the absolute risk of thyroid cancer is still low.[20]

## Summary

All drugs come with side effects and the jabs can affect people in different ways.

- Common side effects include nausea, vomiting, eggy burps, constipation and diarrhoea.
- More serious issues to watch out for (and which require urgent medical attention) include gut paralysis, pancreatitis, gallstones and thyroid cancer. However, we need more high-quality, long-term studies into these risks to get a full understanding.

# CHAPTER 7

# HEALTH BENEFITS OF THE JABS OUTSIDE OF WEIGHT LOSS

When the GLP-1 jabs were first developed, they were assumed to be a single key, tasked with unlocking a single door – to lower blood sugar levels for people with type 2 diabetes. The dramatic weight loss effects have turned out to be an unexpected bonus, and now it seems they may hold the key to other doors. The more we learn, the more we wonder whether these jabs might actually be a master key.

Daniel Drucker, one of the original scientists involved in the discovery of GLP-1 in the 1980s, described it recently as the 'Swiss army knife of metabolism' because, although the drugs were designed to act on GLP-1 receptors in the pancreas, it turns out we have a large number of GLP-1 receptors peppered throughout the body – in the brain, the lungs, heart, stomach and in our blood vessels, too.[1] This could explain how the drug is increasingly displaying unique properties that go beyond its role in controlling blood sugar and weight.[2]

## INFLAMMATION

Acute or short-term inflammation is a natural part of your body's defence and repair mechanism, as a rapid response to infection or injury.

For instance, if you cut yourself, your body will start an inflammatory immune response to help restore and repair the affected area. However, chronic or long-term inflammation is another story. It describes the state of discomfort and mild alert you put your body under when you spend a lifetime smoking, eating an unhealthy diet, or living a sedentary life. It is like a smouldering fire that burns slowly and without flames, making it less noticeable day to day, but very damaging over the long term. The constant stress this low-level inflammation puts on the body can trigger damage throughout the body. Not only does chronic inflammation increase the likelihood of a multitude of health conditions, but it can also speed up the ageing process. It is one of the pillars of accelerated ageing and has even led to scientists coining their own term for it – 'inflammageing'.[3]

Reducing inflammation is a key part of living a healthy lifestyle and can be achieved through switching to a healthy diet and getting lots of good sleep and regular exercise. However, one of the ways the jabs appear to be able to improve our health is through their apparent ability to dampen inflammation throughout the body. We know that high blood-sugar levels can cause inflammation in many areas of the body, including blood vessels, so if GLP-1s improve blood sugar control, they could also be reducing your inflammatory load. Additionally, carrying excess weight and having a poor diet are key contributors to inflammation. Therefore, losing weight (particularly visceral fat) could lead to less inflammation in the body.

The other way they could cause a direct reduction in inflammation is by acting on cells in the immune system. Early studies show that they may help regulate 'pro-inflammatory pathways'.[4] And studies in mice have shown GLP-1s can directly reduce inflammation in the central nervous system.[5]

## HEART DISEASE

A study of more than 17,000 overweight or obese people found an impressive 20 per cent reduction in heart attacks, strokes or death in those taking semaglutide, compared to the placebo group. Interestingly, this reduced risk of heart disease was seen whether the participants lost weight or not. This finding suggests it is not just due to weight loss that the reduction occurs, but that there is another mechanism involved.

Professor John Deanfield, from University College London and the National Institute for Cardiovascular (CV) Outcomes Research (NICOR), who led the study, suggested: 'These alternative mechanisms may include positive impacts on blood sugar, blood pressure, or inflammation, as well as direct effects on the heart muscle and blood vessels, or a combination of one or more of these.'[6]

## KIDNEY FAILURE

Not only do the weight loss medications reduce risk of cardiovascular disease, but they can also reduce kidney complications in patients with type 2 diabetes. In extreme cases, kidney failure can result in a patient requiring dialysis, kidney transplant or death, and almost half of the cases of kidney failure each year occur as a result of complications with type 2 diabetes. But, encouragingly, a recent Novo Nordisk study showed a 24 per cent reduction in kidney disease in patients taking semaglutide compared to the placebo.[7]

However, do we truly know if this reduction in kidney disease and heart disease is due to direct drug-induced 'reduced inflammation', or is it because of the weight loss, and resulting improved metabolic health? Data from the recent 'Look Ahead' study shows that, following a period of intensive lifestyle intervention, participants who were able to achieve any remission of type 2 diabetes (even if it were to return) had a 33 per cent lower rate of chronic kidney disease and a 40 per cent lower rate of cardiovascular disease by the end of a 12-year period! The participants in this study, all of whom had type 2 diabetes, were not taking the weight loss drugs.

## DEMENTIA

Poor metabolic health and obesity substantially increases the risk of dementia. Weight loss, particularly of the more dangerous type of fat called visceral fat that clings to the organs of the body, can help reduce the chance of developing this insidious, dreaded disease. Interestingly, Novo Nordisk, which created Ozempic and Wegovy, is currently conducting trials to see whether GLP-1 can slow the progression of Alzheimer's for those in the early stages of diagnosis.[8]

Doctors now know that chronic, low-grade inflammation in the body can be a pathway to Alzheimer's in people who are susceptible, and it seems inflammation can progressively lead to a loss of neurons (nerve cells found in the brain and nervous system). However, there is some encouraging evidence to suggest that GLP-1 may be able to protect the neurons in the brain. It is thought it may have the potential to reduce nerve cell death, dampen inflammation and increase blood flow to the brain.

## PARKINSON'S DISEASE

The possible 'neuroprotective' features of GLP-1 are the reason why the drug company Novo Nordisk is also investigating whether the drug can be used to treat Parkinson's disease. This is a movement disorder of the nervous system, as suffered by both *Back to the Future* actor Michael J. Fox and boxing legend Muhammad Ali. A small 2013 study involving 46 people with Parkinson's showed positive improvements in activity and movement, as well as improved dementia-rating scales, in those given GLP-1 injections.[9]

## CANCER

GLP-1 drugs are thought to offer some protection against certain cancers. One study compared patients taking metformin (one of the common medications used to reduce blood sugars in people with type 2 diabetes) to those taking GLP-1s as a diabetes treatment between 2005 and 2019. They found that the type 2 diabetics taking the GLP-1 medications saw an impressive 25 per cent reduction in colon cancer.[10] This could be thanks to the way GLP-1 reduces levels of inflammation as it improves blood sugar control and reduces weight. It is known that many cancers have an inflammatory component to them. If reducing obesity reduces the level of inflammation in the body, it may, in turn, help cut your risk of certain cancers.

One contributing factor could also be the way the drug encourages you to eat less. Recent news reports[11] suggest the alarming rise in cases of colon cancer among young people could be caused by our increasingly processed diet. If your diet is made up of predominantly processed foods, reducing your intake will reduce their inflammatory effect on the gut, particularly the colon.

## ADDICTION

One of the most fascinating knock-on effects of the GLP-1 drugs, in my opinion, is their potential role in treating multiple forms of addiction.

With the opioid crisis currently ravaging the US and large parts of Europe, too, any drug that can help addiction is an exciting prospect.

Studies in rats have shown that injecting them with GLP-1s reduces levels of alcohol and drug abuse – it decreased binge drinking and alcohol dependence. Anecdotally, many people taking the jabs have also noticed a decline in other addictive tendencies, from scrolling social media to drinking wine. It is for this reason that there is ongoing research into whether GLP-1s could be used directly to treat addiction to drugs, alcohol and smoking, and not just to ultra-processed junk foods.[12]

A study examining the medical records of over 1 million people in the USA found that those who were taking GLP-1 medications had a 40 per cent reduced chance of overdosing on opioids and, in those with an alcohol addiction, they were 50 per cent less likely to get drunk. This was an observational study and, as such, does not prove causation, but it is interesting nonetheless.

Many elements of modern life are designed for overconsumption because that's what leads to fat profits for the companies supplying these products. From 'doom scrolling' on social media, to gaming, energy drinks, food and even shopping – they are all designed to exploit the reward systems in our brains. Who hasn't found their phone taking over their life? Charter Harley Street Clinical Director and addiction specialist Mandy Saligari once described giving children smartphones as 'giving them a gram of cocaine'.[13]

One large study that looked at our use of mobile phones found that phone and social media use activates the brain's reward centre, and can lead to addiction-like behaviours. The study estimated that more than a quarter of people worldwide fit the criteria of being addicted to their phone.

If GLP-1s can influence or 'dampen' the effect of some of these pathways seen in addiction, perhaps it can change our behaviour and even reduce our phone use?[14]

## KNEE AND HIP REPLACEMENTS

We know that obesity can increase the risk of osteoarthritis by adding to the 'wear and tear' of the joints and cartilage, but is also hikes the levels of general inflammation throughout the body. In a trial of patients given semaglutide (Ozempic), the participants not only lost 14 per cent of their body weight but, compared to a placebo, they saw a significant improvement in their symptoms of pain from osteoarthritis.[15] In fact, other studies have found that those taking GLP-1 medications were less likely to need knee replacements than those not taking these drugs.[16]

I spoke to Professor Roy Taylor, Professor of Medicine and Metabolism at Newcastle University, who believes one area where weight loss medications could have potential is in helping people lose weight to better prepare them for joint replacement surgery. This could both minimise their risk of complications in the operating theatre and maximise their chance of recovery afterwards.

'Having surgery when you are an optimal weight can reduce your chance of pain, suffering and potential complications, not to mention the number of days you might need to stay at hospital,' he told me. 'It offers hope to people who might have been refused an operation because they are overweight.'

The outcomes for those about to go under the knife to have their knee or hip replaced are currently far worse if that person is carrying a lot of weight, and are very poor if they are severely obese. As a result, many NHS orthopaedic surgeons will not perform an operation until that person has lost weight. The jabs could offer an effective boost to people who are rendered immobile and in pain by their joint problems, and who might struggle to lose weight in any other way. Losing weight in these circumstances would reduce anaesthetic risks, improve recovery and potentially extend the life of a joint replacement from five to 20 years.

## BIPOLAR AND SCHIZOPHRENIA

As a doctor I have worked in the psychiatric departments of different hospitals and I have seen how the anti-psychotic medication given to people with bipolar, schizophrenia or severe depression can lead to a huge amount of weight gain and dramatically increase the risk of type 2 diabetes. This is likely a contributing factor to the fact that, on average, the life expectancy of people with schizophrenia is a full 15 years shorter than 'normal' life expectancy.

In the world of psychiatry, these weight loss medications could help stave off excess weight gain and reduce the risks of developing type 2 diabetes, improving quality of life, too.

## DEPRESSION

Some people report weight gain when taking anti-depressants, and depression and anxiety are more than twice as common in people with type 2 diabetes. Although there were initial concerns about an increased risk of suicidal thoughts when taking these weight loss drugs, as we've seen in Chapter 6, it appears the opposite is more likely to be true. Recent studies have shown the use of the GLP-1 semaglutide and tirzepatide is associated with a lower risk of depression and anxiety.[17]

When I spoke to Adele, a health-care worker working in an inpatient psychiatry unit who was taking tirzepatide (Mounjaro), she told me she feels a lot happier and more confident: 'I think my mood's improved a lot. It's like I've had a mood boost.'

## SLEEP APNOEA

Weight loss medications have great potential as a treatment for obstructive sleep apnoea (OSA), which is a condition where your breathing stops for 10 seconds or more, often multiple times, during the night. This is caused when the muscles in your throat and tongue relax and temporarily block your airway, putting undue strain on your heart, and leaving you feeling very tired the next day.

My dad, Michael, was a chronic insomniac. During middle-age he had steadily piled on the pounds, as many people do. As his weight increased, so did his snoring. If you were sleeping in the room next to him, it felt like an earthquake going through the house at times (my poor mum). After losing more than 9kg in 2012, and keeping it off, his snoring went almost completely away. Whenever his weight crept up even a little bit, the snoring would return (though fortunately less ferocious than before).

Not everyone who snores has sleep apnoea, but it is associated with it. For every 10 per cent increase in body weight, your risk of OSA increases sixfold, but it is frequently a 'hidden' diagnosis, as it presents in ways that would not be obvious to most people. One Swedish study estimated that as many as 20 per cent of women have OSA, 90 per cent of whom do not know they have it. You may have a partner who prods you in the night to encourage you to gasp for breath, but classic signs include falling asleep watching TV, or while sitting in the cinema or theatre, when you are the passenger in a car or even while sitting and talking to someone.[18]

In severe OSA, your airway can collapse more than 30 times in an hour while you sleep. A loud snoring sound is made each time your breathing returns. As you can imagine, regularly cutting off oxygen to your brain and body is not a good thing. OSA can increase the risk of stroke and high blood pressure.

The 'gold standard' of treatment is a CPAP machine – a device like a gas mask that is placed over your face and which pumps air into your lungs as you sleep. However, because 70 per cent of sufferers are obese, weight loss is the first line treatment for mild OSA.[19] In the future, GLP-1s could be used as a direct treatment, given how much difference weight loss can make to the symptoms of OSA.

## LIVER DISEASE

Another 'hidden disease' is non-alcoholic fatty liver disease (NAFLD), which is caused not by alcohol, but by carrying excess weight and having a poor diet. I say it is a 'hidden disease' because recent studies estimate an astonishing third of the world's population now suffers from NAFLD, but the vast majority will not be aware they have it.

NAFLD can increase the risk of poor metabolic health, including type 2 diabetes. In its most severe form, it can cause scarring and impairment of the liver (cirrhosis) or even liver failure. Those with NAFLD also have a higher risk of heart disease, strokes and liver cancer.

Most cases of NAFLD can be resolved by losing between 10–15 per cent of body weight, especially in those living with obesity, which means GLP-1s could be used as a direct treatment of NAFLD in the future.[20]

## Summary

- The weight loss jabs could have numerous health benefits outside of weight loss.

- It turns out that the drugs designed to act on GLP-1 receptors in the pancreas (to stimulate the production of insulin) also act on the GLP-1 receptors throughout the body – in the brain, lungs, heart, stomach and blood vessels.

- There is a possibility that GLP-1 medication reduces levels of chronic inflammation throughout the body, which is responsible for many of the diseases of ageing.

- The jabs could reduce the risk of heart disease, kidney failure, dementia, Parkinson's disease and certain cancers.

- The jabs could play an interesting potential role in the control of addiction.

- They could help patients lose weight before joint replacement surgery, prevent weight gain from anti-depressants and anti-psychotic medication, and help those who suffer from sleep apnoea (OSA) and people with unknown fatty liver disease.

# PART 3

# THE NEW WAY TO LOSE WEIGHT

I'm deeply concerned that in the mad rush to get hold of weight loss jabs people aren't getting the advice they need and they're not thinking carefully enough about the longer-term implications: how do you know when to increase or decrease your dose? What happens when you reach your target weight? Can you afford to stay on the jabs forever? How do you feel about the fact that there are no studies to show what impact these jabs might have on your long-term health?

It's a difficult path to tread, but I am confident this book will help you navigate it.

To gain the most you can out of the weight loss medications, you can't just stick a needle in your tummy and hope for the best. Dietary and lifestyle support is crucial. The jabs can be an extremely effective tool in your tool box, but they are not the only tool. To create long-lasting changes in habits, including an improved diet and integrating activity and exercise into your life, you must have a plan in place even before you start taking the jabs. You'll reduce your risk of malnutrition, you'll hang on to precious muscle, and protect yourself against future frailty.

This is also how you improve your chances of keeping the weight off in the future.

In this important section of the book, I will outline the safest ways to take these weight loss drugs, the best ways to eat to maximise your nutritional input, and I will explain how you can protect your muscles when you are taking the jabs and in the long-term.

This section culminates with a simple but powerfully effective three-stage plan to guide you safely through your weight loss journey and to support you in maintaining your optimal weight and your health long into the future.

I am hopeful that most people will not need to be on these drugs for life but will use them to kick-start a healthy weight loss journey. If you strive to make improvements in your diet, focusing on eating real and filling nutritious foods, and exercising regularly, the weight loss jabs can find a healthy place in the mix.

# CHAPTER 8

# HOW TO USE THE WEIGHT LOSS DRUGS SAFELY

In an ideal world, these powerful weight loss drugs would only be prescribed by a qualified and experienced health worker, who would give nutritional advice and who would be on hand to offer guidance and support through your weight loss journey. Sadly only a few premium-priced private clinics offer this kind of service, and most people are self-prescribing and taking them without an instruction manual.

In the original studies in which participants lost more than 15 per cent of their body weight taking Ozempic, they also received significant 'lifestyle interventions', which included a prescribed, reduced-calorie diet, increased physical activity and monthly counselling by qualified health professionals. But today, very few people are getting this level of service.

Despite my extensive research into this subject I am not in a position to tell anyone how they should or shouldn't use the injections, and the best advice I can offer is the sort of thing your GP might say. If you are thinking about taking them, you should speak to a health professional in the first instance. Your GP may not be able to prescribe weight loss jabs, even if you do fit the NICE (National Institute of Clinical Excellence) guidelines criteria (a BMI over 27 with a weight-related health condition, or a BMI over 30), but they will have access to your medical records and can advise if they suspect potential complications or a need for close monitoring. Informing your GP means they will be better equipped to offer support further down the line, if you do source the drugs privately and come unstuck.

## DO YOU REALLY NEED THE JABS?

Before you go rushing in, please ask yourself whether you really want to rely on drugs or whether a good diet would work just as well? Could you cope with the probability of nausea and the possibility of vomiting? Few drugs come without side effects. Aiming for a drug-free life is generally a better choice. Don't think of taking them for weight loss purposes, if you're not really quite overweight. These drugs are licensed privately as a weight loss aid for anyone with a BMI over 27 and at least one weight-related complication. Their safety cannot be guaranteed outside of this licensing window. Most private clinics will ask you to send a recent photo, a photo of your scales and your passport in a bid to verify that you are overweight.

## CAN YOU GET THEM ON THE NHS?

Probably not. In the UK, you might be prescribed GLP-1 medications if you have type 2 diabetes, but you are extremely unlikely to get it on the NHS for weight loss alone. Official NICE guidelines in the UK state the jabs can be prescribed, free, to people with a BMI over 30 (27.5 for some ethnic groups) with at least one life-limiting, weight-related health condition, such as high blood pressure, diabetes or heart disease. But in practice, even if you qualify, you're unlikely to get the jabs on the NHS.

Right now, even if your GP does think jabs might be helpful for you, you will only be able to get an NHS prescription if your GP refers you to an NHS weight-management specialist. These services are underfunded and overstretched and your chances of seeing a specialist is a bit of a postcode lottery. The Obesity Health Alliance (OHA) published a recent report that found that people frequently have to wait three to five years to be seen by weight loss services. In fact, some services are even closed to new referrals as demand far exceeds their capacity.[1]

## DO YOUR HOMEWORK

If you are considering a private clinic, look for one that offers support and lifestyle advice. Check the clinic has been inspected by the Care Quality Commission for safety, www.cqc.org.uk. Only use a registered pharmacy (identified by a green cross badge next to the words Registered Pharmacy and a registration number, or you can check they're registered at www.pharmacyregulation.org). If there's no physical address or phone number, and if you can't call and ask questions, probably best not to buy from them. Reputable pharmacies will ask you to fill in online forms about your weight, medical history and any current medications you are taking, and you may be asked to upload pictures. This information will be reviewed by doctors to see if you meet the criteria set out in the drug's licence.

---

### Beware of fake jabs

Whenever a craze like weight loss medication takes off, there are also likely to be 'sharks' and scammers circling the waters, ready to take advantage of unfortunate victims by selling counterfeit

---

medications. Sadly, there are now hundreds of websites selling fake versions of the weight loss drugs[2] – they might take the form of syringe pens that contain the wrong dose, pens that contain no active ingredient and pens containing actively harmful and dangerous ingredients.

The concern about counterfeit GLP-1s has become so great that the World Health Organization (WHO) has issued a global alert about the problem. In the UK, the drugs regulator has seized shipments of counterfeit batches of the drugs.[3]

Drug company Eli Lilly is currently in a legal battle with a Washington-based firm selling do-it-yourself GLP-1 kits. You do not need a doctor's referral or even a prescription for these kits, which come with written instructions for creating a sterile solution from a white powder. The product is stamped: 'A research chemical for lab research and veterinary purposes only', yet the company offers advice on how to inject it with a needle.[4]

## START LOW AND GO SLOW

Medications like the GLP-1s should be taken by slowly 'titrating' the dose to find the level that suits you over a period of weeks and months. Your decision on how high to take the dose will depend on the speed of weight loss you need, but also the severity of the side effects you might be experiencing. Titration is a standard procedure with almost all medications and is normally done with the support of a doctor. However, in the 'Wild West' of the GLP-1 world this is rarely the case.

Currently, standard practice is to increase the dose gradually in increments each month until you find the dose that keeps your appetite in check without side effects, then to stay on that dose until you reach your target weight or indefinitely.

I have spoken to many people who were encouraged by online pharmacies to increase the dose (and therefore the cost) continuously, despite suffering severe side effects. Mental-health worker Adele told me she was advised to increase her dose of Mounjaro from 5mg to 7.5mg. 'I'd eat a meal, then I'd vomit. Then I'd vomit in the morning as well . . . so I've gone back down to the lower dose,' she says.

My mother's GP friend Anya, who works in a deprived inner-city area, told a similar story of her experience with patients starting the GLP-1 drugs: 'Everyone seems to ramp up the dose very quickly, and I don't understand that! Maybe the drugs companies or online pharmacies encourage it because they get more money . . . the higher dose is more expensive.'

Some people might find a lower dose is enough. Everyone reacts differently. It is rarely a good idea to leap up the dosage, because that's when the problematic and potentially dangerous side effects really kick in.

## FIND YOUR SWEET SPOT

You may find the lowest dose works for a month or two before food noise starts creeping back and weight loss dwindles, making you feel compelled to increase the dose. However, at the moment there is not much evidence to suggest you develop a tolerance or become desensitised to the GLP-1 drugs. Our digestive tracts do appear to show some tolerance to certain symptoms from the drugs over time, so nausea can lessen, but this is even more of a reason to start the medications on a low dose and only slowly increase.

Like most medications, there is a surprisingly large amount of individual variability in response, which can depend on environment and genetics, as well as diet and lifestyle. For instance, you may notice a rise in hunger levels if you start exercising frequently, or if you go through a period of eating processed food. Protein and fibre are more filling than refined carbohydrates, which the body burns through rapidly, causing blood sugar spikes that can leave you feeling hungry shortly afterwards.

Weight loss can sometimes begin to level off when you reach a 'healthy weight', whether you are on or off the weight loss drugs, as other hormones are released to reignite your appetite once more. This is explained by a concept called 'set point theory', where your body sets its own weight range and then attempts to maintain this weight at all costs. So, your body might fight back in an attempt to prevent further depletion of your fat stores by slowing your metabolic rate, increasing your ghrelin levels (the hunger hormone) and prompting cravings to encourage you to eat more. Not only can ghrelin increase hunger but it also can affect the reward centres in the brain and encourage us to seek out calorie-dense foods.

## WHEN AND HOW DO YOU STOP TAKING THE JABS?

The big question faced by anyone taking or thinking about taking one of the weight loss jabs is not whether they'll work – they have been shown to enable impressively swift and significant weight loss – but whether you'll be able to keep the weight off after you stop taking them.

Alarmingly, studies show two-thirds of the weight is regained by the end of first year off the drugs.[5] A clinical trial funded by the makers of tirzepatide (Mounjaro) gave participants prepackaged meals and diet and exercise advice with their weekly injections and found they lost an average of 21 per cent of their body weight over three months. But when some of those participants were switched to a placebo jab, they regained 14 per cent of their body weight.[6] The results were similar when participants were given semaglutide (Wegovy) followed by a placebo.[7]

Clearly these medications can enable huge levels of weight loss, but when you stop taking them, the weight creeps back. This is worrying because of the likelihood that the weight you regain could be mostly fat, and not the muscle you are likely to have lost. This means your post-jab body composition could be worse off than when you started the drug, with damaging implications for your long-term health, including an increased risk of frailty or poor metabolic health.

I suspect the drugs companies would love you to continue taking the jabs for ever, but that's prohibitively expensive for most people and, besides, you can't ignore the fact that there haven't been long-term studies to show whether these jabs at the higher weight loss dose could be affecting other aspects of your health in frightening ways. Although GLP-1s have been used – in very small doses – by people with type 2 diabetes for almost 20 years, the higher weight loss dose has only been in use since 2021, so we just don't know what the downstream consequences might be.

Younger people who are starting the drugs now may end up taking the higher dose for decades.

A recent report by Reuters found that only one in four people are still taking semaglutide – Ozempic or Wegovy – two years after starting it.[8] This could be due to the high costs (in the USA a course of injections was priced at $1,500 a month for some time). Prices have dropped (in the UK you can start on a low dose of Mounjaro for around £150 a month, but the cost rises with the dose), which means people might decide to keep taking these drugs for extended periods of time, if they can afford to do so. Some people are stopped by the side effects, which can intensify as the dose increases, and others by a desire to go back to a 'normal' pattern of eating.

Dr David Unwin told me: 'Compliance can start to be a problem when people get sick of not enjoying their food as much. I've noticed some people start having little holidays from the drugs. And they say, well, it's Christmas. I want to enjoy my food . . . and then they start having longer breaks.'

## WILL THE FOOD NOISE RETURN?

Unfortunately, yes. When people start the weight loss medications, many describe how the food noise vanishes, meaning hunger and the urge to eat is no longer a dominant part of their lives. The weight loss drugs act like soundproof ear defenders to block out the extra food noise. However, when the medication is stopped, those ear defenders are removed and the food noise returns, just as loud as ever. Your appetite can return with a vengeance.

Domenica Rubino, Director of the Washington Center for Weight Management and Research, is one of many scientists who worry that the

GLP-1s only put a temporary sticking plaster on dysregulated appetite signalling. 'I try to explain that these are chronic medications, but I think everybody secretly feels, "Yeah, but you know what, I'm different, and once I hit my weight goal, I'll be okay." But the reality is, the brain is quite powerful,' he says.[9]

Some, like Dr Martin Whyte, an Associate Professor of Metabolic Medicine at the University of Surrey, worry that because the doses of GLP-1s are far greater than the body would naturally expect to receive, they may suppress the body's ability to secrete GLP-1 on its own. As a result, people's hunger may return even more voraciously when they stop taking the jabs.

Tanya, a retired GP with an interest in weight loss and obesity, took Mounjaro while following The Fast 800 programme and, although she did reach her weight loss goal, she, like many I spoke to, was anxious about stopping the medication. 'I'm thinking, what do I do next time? What happens if I can't control my weight? It's scary. When the hunger returns it does feel a bit like withdrawal. You think, "Oh no, I'm hungry. Oh dear, I'll put all the weight back on again and end up in exactly the same position as I was by next year."'

The reality today is that many people will have purchased their medications via an online pharmacist, most of whom offer limited support and advice about how to live and what to eat when you're on the jabs, let alone when you stop taking them. The obesogenic food environment we live in remains the same, our habits remain the same, our cooking remains the same . . . and, inevitably, many people will go on to regain a large portion of the weight they've lost.

It is interesting that the dating app Hinge states it is 'Designed to be deleted', which refers to its alleged aim to match people with the perfect romantic partner so they no longer need the app. It would be great if the same could be said for weight loss jabs. The ultimate aim would be to stop taking them entirely or, at the very least, to titrate the medication right down so the lowest possible dose keeps you on the straight and narrow. But, unless you simultaneously change your lifestyle, this quest is virtually impossible. As you remove the ear defenders, the food noise returns. However, changes to your lifestyle and habits can at the very least work as effective ear plugs.

---

### Can you 'microdose'?

Some people are choosing to stay on a low dose permanently to avoid relapses, and clinical trials are being planned to assess whether a 'maintenance dose', which comes with fewer side effects, can be prescribed on a long-term basis. Some doctors are offering a bespoke service of supervised 'microdosing' of weight loss jabs.[10] This means playing with a very low starter dose (2.5mg of Mounjaro or even just 0.25mg of Ozempic) and offering a booster dose when needed. This is popular in the USA and available at some private clinics in the UK for about £250 a month. There is talk of people 'hacking' their dose by taking less than prescribed or prolonging their pens by injecting less often (every other week, or one week each month). But you should never do this without medical supervision.

---

## TAKING THE DRUG IF YOU AREN'T OVERWEIGHT

At the moment, the big pharma companies are shipping out as much of the drug as they can. Inevitably, not everyone who is taking it will fit the guidelines. And, certainly, many people are taking the drugs as a quick-fix without changing their lifestyles.

I had a chat with a woman in her thirties, who wished to remain anonymous, who was able to get once-weekly GLP-1 medications via the beauticians she attends. She was able to get the medication despite not fulfilling the guidelines: 'Someone submitted the application on my behalf. I said I didn't want my GP to know – all completely off the radar.'

Another person told me: 'Everyone's on it now. Even skinny people are on it.'

This drug was not intended for people with a BMI in the healthy range, which is between 18.5 and 25, and it does concern me that people are able to access the medications through online pharmacies, which means they do have the potential to be abused by people living with anorexia or eating disorders. The safety and risks of these drugs have only been studied in an overweight or obese population. They certainly shouldn't provide a quick fix for people just wanting to lose an extra couple of kilos for their next beach holiday. When used for the wrong purposes, the risks are greater.

Lottie Moss is the younger half-sister of English supermodel Kate Moss and also a fashion model. She spoke on her 'Dream On' podcast about using Ozempic to drop from 60kg to 53kg and warned her listeners of the potential dangers of taking the drug: 'I felt so sick one day, I said to my friend, "I can't keep any water down. I can't keep any food down, no liquids, nothing. I need to go to the hospital. I feel really sick."

'The amount that I was taking was for people who were 100 kilos and over, and I'm in the 50 kilos range,' she added. 'It's these small things I wish I'd known before taking it.

'I literally had a seizure from how dehydrated I was, which honestly was the scariest thing that's ever happened to me in my life.'[11]

---

### Case study

Some people find weight loss drugs useful to kickstart a healthier lifestyle. That's the case with Pawel, an A&E consultant based in the northwest. As a doctor, he was aware his weight was putting his health at risk, so he started using a GLP-1 weight loss medication:

'My weight had been creeping up little by little each year and, by the time I reached 150kg, I started getting minor infections, weird skin issues and my legs started swelling, which had never happened in the past.

'The leaflets issued with the jabs were disappointing. They were very colourful, informing me that I'd be eating less and, if I felt sick, I should eat more carbohydrates. But there wasn't a single sentence about how long to take the drug (it just said a minimum of six months) and no plan for coming off. I was very sceptical – it was as if they wanted me to keep taking it for ever.

---

'So, after four or five months, I decided to taper off the dose, gradually weaning myself off it. I very closely monitored my hunger signals and cravings, and ate healthily, following The Fast 800 principles. By intermittent fasting – sticking to 800 calories a few days a week and eating normal food a few days a week, but cutting right down on carbohydrates – for a year or so, I lost as much weight after coming off Saxenda as I had when I was taking the jabs: 60kg in total.'

## HOW TO STOP SAFELY

As far as we know, it is unlikely to be dangerous to stop taking the jabs abruptly. You shouldn't experience any kind of withdrawal. However, you are likely to notice 'food noise' rushing back. This is why pairing it with a good food programme and focusing on lifestyle changes is so vitally important.

If you have successfully lost weight, you may feel some anxiety or stress about stopping the medication, so tapering down the medication may be a preferable way to stop.

Clearly this approach is only relevant if you are taking the medication for weight loss rather than type 2 diabetes. If in any doubt, speak to your healthcare provider for advice.

## DON'T RELY ON THE DRUGS
## TO DO ALL THE WORK FOR YOU

Dr David Unwin speaks for many medics when he says: 'We all want to continue eating cake and junk food – some of us are addicted to these foods. And these weight loss jabs seem to be providing a remedy. But what happens when you stop taking them? Haven't you just kicked the can along the road? Isn't the problem still there? Because you haven't addressed the actual reason that people overeat and gain weight. It isn't good enough just to give people these injections and then walk away,' he told me. 'What you've got there is a possible opportunity to learn to live your life differently.'

I couldn't agree more.

If you do decide to try the jabs, it is important to make a few changes before you start taking them. Commit to switching to a healthy diet and regular exercise, and make a long-term plan for when the drug will be stopped. Use the opportunity provided by the drugs, which shrink your appetite, to reset your approach to your diet and lifestyle.

In the following pages I'll show you how.

## Summary

- Talk to your GP or a healthcare provider about whether weight loss jabs might be suitable and appropriate for you.
- The weight loss dose of the jabs is only licensed for people with a BMI over 27 and are suffering from at least one obesity-related condition (such as type 2 diabetes or heart disease) or who have a BMI over 30 (classified as 'obese').

- As of the end of 2024, even if you qualify for treatment on the NHS, you are unlikely to be able to get the jabs. Most people find a reputable pharmacy or clinic. If you do opt to start the medication, look for one that offers diet and lifestyle support.
- When you start, it would be sensible to begin on a lower dose and only increase it very slowly if your weight loss stalls (don't be tempted to ramp up the dose).
- Never rely on the drugs to do all the work for you – you must eat healthily and exercise regularly.

# CHAPTER 9

# STAYING NOURISHED – HOW TO EAT WELL ON AND OFF THE WEIGHT LOSS DRUGS

Whether you are thinking about taking weight loss medication, you are actually on the jabs, you're tapering off your dose, or you're trying desperately hard to maintain your new weight having finished taking the drugs, you must eat good, real food.

These weight loss drugs will drastically reduce your appetite and can substantially restrict the quantity of food you are eating. Losing weight, if your metabolic health is poor, can be very beneficial to your health. But if we want to live happy, healthy and long lives, we need to make sure we are not just restricting ourselves, but also eating a complete and varied diet, too. Food is and should continue to be a delight for the tastebuds, body and brain.

With my family background, you probably won't be surprised to hear me sing the praises of a Mediterranean-style diet. It is a science-backed, nutritional health-bullet that my dad passionately believed in and which my mum continues to put into practice. It is how we should all be eating – whether on the jabs or off.

When we think of the Mediterranean, we might imagine a country such as Italy. And when we think of Italian food, many of us immediately think of pasta and pizza. But the traditional, Mediterranean-style diet is one that consists of plenty of olive oil, whole grains, vegetables, nuts and seeds, as well as seafood, oily fish, some dairy and chicken in moderation, as well as the occasional glass of red wine. It emphasises smaller amounts of red meat, but does not exclude it completely. The true Mediterranean-style diet is highly nutritious. It is one of the most researched diets in the world, and has the most evidence supporting it as a healthy dietary pattern. Following such a diet is a great way to maximise your nutrition while you are losing weight, and help you beat the odds and keep the weight off when you stop taking the jabs.

When researchers compared a Mediterranean diet infused with extra-virgin olive oil and nuts against a low-fat diet with plenty of pasta, potatoes and rice, they found those on the higher fat Mediterranean diet saw a 30 per cent reduction in heart attacks and stroke, a 58 per cent reduced risk of type 2 diabetes, a 51 per cent less chance of breast cancer and reduced cognitive decline. In the study, those following the Mediterranean-style diet were encouraged to eat olive oil, nuts, fresh fruit and vegetables, legumes, white meat such as chicken (instead of red meat), fatty fish and seafood. Interestingly, this group were even encouraged to drink at least one glass of wine a day. This Mediterranean-style diet produced far better health outcomes than those following a low-fat diet.[1]

The results were phenomenal, and the trial was stopped over a year early due to the clear magnitude of benefits emerging from those following the Mediterranean-style diet. Fascinatingly, research has begun to show that it can improve our mood, too – which makes healthy eating a positive and enriching experience, even when you're trying to lose weight.

Professor Felice Jacka is a professor of Nutritional Psychiatry and founder of the Food and Mood Centre at Deakin University in Melbourne. Through the SMILES study, she and her team were aiming to look at the impact of a Mediterranean-style diet on depression. When efforts were made to recruit patients for the trial, she found it difficult, as she did not have the support of psychiatrists or doctors. She suspected this was because the medical establishment felt it was unlikely that dietary changes would make a great deal of difference. But, once she got going, she placed one group of people who had been diagnosed with depression on a Mediterranean-style diet. The people in this group were also asked to reduce their consumption of UPFs, including sweets, refined cereals, fried food, fast food, processed meats and sugary drinks, and to increase their consumption of whole foods. For instance, replacing processed cereals with unprocessed oats, swapping white bread for sourdough, and switching pizzas for stir-fries.

The control group was encouraged to stick to its familiar diet, but it received extra counselling sessions. The results were startling. Those in the group following the modified Mediterranean diet saw a significant reduction in their depression scores. In fact, 32 per cent of that group saw a remission of their depression, compared to just 8 per cent of the control group.

The study highlighted how important the quality of our diet is for mood, whether those involved lost weight or not. The closer the participants stuck to a less processed, Mediterranean-style diet, the more their depression improved.[2]

I discussed the fascinating SMILES study in more depth with Professor Felice Jacka, who highlighted how important a quality diet, rich in nutrients, is: 'The SMILES diet was not a weight loss diet and people didn't lose weight, and yet they experienced a very, very powerful benefit to their moderate to severe clinical depression.' She continued, 'And so our point when we're talking about diet quality is forget about your body size. It's not about that; it's about how you nurture your body's systems, how you nurture your gut and the microbiome, how you nurture your brain, how you nurture it all. Your immune system in particular – all of these things are influenced by the *quality* of what you eat.'

Several studies since this groundbreaking work have shown supporting evidence that following a Mediterranean-style diet can indeed be beneficial to our mental wellbeing. This includes a randomised control trial last year that showed reduced anxiety, depression and stress in the group assigned to following a Mediterranean-style diet.[3]

Fortunately, the principles of the Mediterranean-style diet can be applied to multiple other cuisines – from Chinese to Indian to Mexican. One country renowned for its population's long life expectancy is Japan. A traditional Japanese diet shares many similarities with a Mediterranean diet: it contains large amounts of fresh vegetables, legumes and plenty of oily fish or seaweed. Both these diets are highly nutritious, containing plenty of vitamins, minerals and fibre, as well as important fats such as omega-3.

If you eventually stop the weight loss medications, it is far more likely that you will regain the lost weight if you have not changed your diet. The Mediterranean diet is an excellent long-term option, as it provides foods that are filling, as well as good for the body. It has foods that contain a great range of satiating protein, fibre and healthy fats, which makes it easier to keep the weight within a healthy range for the long term.

All the recipes at the back of this book are based on the principles of the Mediterranean-style diet, so you can't go wrong by incorporating some of them into your regular meals.

## Eat like a Sardinian

Sardinia is the second largest island in Italy. With its white, sandy beaches, rugged coves and emerald-blue water, it is an immensely picturesque island in the Mediterranean. Not only is Sardinia a place of great natural beauty, it is also a region marked by an unusually large number of centenarians. *Per capita* there are 10 times as many people living over the age of 100 years as in the US.[4] Perdasdefogu, a remote town in the mountains of Sardinia, holds the world record for the highest concentration of centenarians in one region.[5] Isolated by the mountains and away from the clutches of modern life, many Sardinians in these regions have been able to maintain a more traditional diet. The elderly residents of the town put their impressive longevity down to a number of factors, including their simple diet of fresh whole foods, their continuous movement and physical activity, and their strong social bonds and sense of community.

Adolfo Melis, a resident of Perdasdefogu, is one of nine siblings in the village who hold the record for the oldest siblings in the world.

He is a youthful 98 years old and thinks diet is an important reason why his siblings have seen such longevity: 'Everything we ate came from the garden. What you put into your stomach is so important – if you abuse the stomach, it doesn't resist.'[6]

The *Guardian* reported in 2022 about the latest resident of Perdasdefogu to join this elite group of centenarians – a man called Vittorio Lai, nicknamed 'Pistol'. Vittorio was pictured standing proudly in his flat cap, bow tie and suit, next to a sign reading *'Perdasdefogu Record Mondiale della longevita familiare'* (Persdasdefogu World Record for family longevity) to mark the achievement. At the age of 100, Vittorio still drives and hunts wild boar. It appears that in Perdasdefogu, being 100 is the new 80!

## MAX OUT ON PLANT-BASED FOODS

The Mediterranean diet is renowned for its health benefits, largely because it emphasises eating an abundance of vegetables, fruits and other essential components for wellbeing, such as plant-based fibre, beans, lentils, chickpeas and whole grains.

Currently the UK recommendation for daily fibre intake is 30g per day. Yet as few as 1 in 10 people are getting enough of this excellent gut-friendly substance. If you start taking weight loss drugs and you don't improve your low-fibre diet, you will be depleting your fibre consumption even more. You'll be in danger of cutting out what little fibre remains in your diet.

The focus on fibre is even more important because one of the unfortunate side effects of the GLP-1s is constipation. This is partly because the drugs slow down the movement of food through the digestive tract, but also because generally there is a lack of fibre in the diet. The reality is that we *all* should be aiming to eat far more fibre, but this is even more important if you are taking GLP-1s.

Fibre helps bulk out our stool in our gut, making it easier for it to pass through and absorb more water. Another handy benefit of having plenty of fibre in our diets, is that it can leave us feeling full for longer and reduce blood sugar spikes. This helps us on the weight loss journey.

## FEED YOUR MICROBIOME

Constipation is only one part of the story. If you're not eating enough fibre, you could also be starving your gut microbiome. This is the populations of trillions of microorganisms that live in the gut. The microbiome contains a diverse range of different microbes, such as bacteria, yeast, viruses and fungi, that influence us just as much as we influence them. This vast array of gut flora weighs as much as our brains, a mighty 2kg. There are the same number of bacteria in our intestines as there are cells in the human body. We are half bacteria, half body.

It is like a rainforest which has its own ecosystem teeming with life. When a tropical rainforest has its perfect climate – warm but not too hot, plenty of rainfall and a rich forest floor – its biodiversity will flourish. However, changes to climate or other outside forces, including man-made interferences, can cause significant damage to the flora and balance of the rainforest habitat So, too, for our microbiome.

What is the optimum 'climate' for our microbiome? For a start, having fibre present is essential. Fibre is not broken down by our stomachs, so it reaches our gut without being fully digested. Once there, the bacteria in our gut feasts on the fibre, breaking it down, and the microbes get busy working in the dark reaches of the intestines to produce lots of highly beneficial byproducts. The most important of these are short chain fatty acids (SCFAs), which provide us with an array of great health benefits for both the body and the brain. They also help maintain the gut wall. If you don't eat enough fibre, fewer SCFAs will be produced and the gut lining becomes weakened, which can lead to a 'leaky gut'. Having a leaky gut can allow toxins, microbes and other substances to breach the gut wall, causing inflammation throughout the body. In the brain, SCFAs help regulate our mood and their anti-inflammatory properties help reduce the risk of neurodegenerative diseases such as Alzheimer's or Parkinson's.

We also now know that a high-fibre diet can reduce your risk of cancer and cardiovascular disease. The alarming rise of colorectal cancer among young people could be, at least partly, linked to the fact that our fibre intake is far below the recommended guidelines. The best way to get fibre in your diet and encourage a happy, diverse population of gut microbes is to eat plant-based, whole foods, such as legumes (beans, lentils, chickpeas) and whole grains, such as oats (when minimally processed). Other good whole foods include cabbage, avocado, spinach, berries, apples, nuts and seeds. Remember that ultra-processed junk foods are generally lacking in fibre because it is often removed to improve shelf life and palatability.

If your portion size has shrunk dramatically on the weight loss jabs and you are not focusing on fibre, it is very likely that you could be starving your microbiome and stopping it from effectively fulfilling all the functions it is designed to do.

## Eat a rainbow

Aim to eat the widest possible variety of types and colours of fruit and vegetables you can find. The rainbow colours of plants indicate that they have a proliferation of 'phytochemicals', which are compounds designed to protect the plant from predators, such as insects, or sunshine and disease. When eaten by us, these phytochemicals (or phytonutrients) have a similarly protective effect. Having a good range of different phytonutrients also helps feed and proliferate the populations of beneficial gut microbiota, while limiting the growth of 'bad' bacteria. Phytonutrients are important antioxidants – they help mop up and neutralise unstable molecules called free radicals. These antioxidants help prevent damage to cells, limiting the effects of ageing and reducing the risk of diseases, like cancer and heart disease. Eating the same beige food day in and day out will severely limit the range of foods and nutrients your body receives. So aim for a range of colours.

**Green:** fill your plate with leafy greens (kale, spinach, lettuce) and brassicas (broccoli, cabbage, Brussels sprouts and cauliflower). These nutrient-dense green vegetables provide anti-inflammatory and cancer-blocking properties.

**Yellow and orange:** these colours signal 'carotenoids' and are found in sweet potato, butternut squash, tomatoes, peppers, egg yolks and melons.

**White:** phytochemical rich and microbiome friendly, white foods include garlic, onions, shallots and leeks.

**Purple:** rich in 'flavonoids', a range of evidence suggests that purple foods are anti-inflammatory, cardio-protective and neuro-protective.[7] So tuck into dark chocolate, black tea, red wine, aubergines, dark red apples, grapes, blackberries and blueberries.

## THE GUT-BRAIN CONNECTION

It may not be able to complete a crossword, write a song or solve complex algebra, yet the nervous system in the gut, or the enteric nervous system (ENS), is often referred to as a 'second brain'. In fact, it has the same number of neurons as your average cat.

The brain is in constant communication with our gut and when we treat our gut well, the two are good friends. Not only does the central nervous system (CNS) and brain send signals to the gut, but the gut sends signals back. This 'gut–brain axis' communication happens with the help of a range of hormones, neurotransmitters, neurons and other chemical-signalling molecules.

When we receive shocking or upsetting news, we may find it 'gut wrenching'. And, of course, when we follow our intuition we are said to be 'going with our gut'. It is the only region of the body with its own complete and complex nervous system, and which can operate independently from the central nervous system.[8]

We can have more influence on this great gut–brain friendship than many might think. Some of what we eat is food for us, to keep our body's engine running. But some of what we eat is food for our gut; for our microbiome.

## GET FERMENTING

The bacteria in our gut feed on fibre and this 'prebiotic' substance helps the microbes thrive and multiply. But if you want to increase the diversity of your gut microbiome, you need to be eating 'probiotic' foods, which contain live microorganisms, as well. A great source of these is fermented foods, such as yoghurt, cheese, sauerkraut, kombucha and kimchi – and even dark chocolate counts! My mum, Clare, is a big fan of making probiotic ferments, so her fridge has a shelf of purple sauerkraut, kimchi and other tasty, fermented foods, and she aims to eat fermented foods four or five times a day. And the billions of microbes in her gut love it, too.

Humans have been fermenting food for thousands of years. Making yoghurt has long been a practice across Europe and the Middle East, and not just because it helps the milk last longer. Different fermented foods originate in different regions – from kimchi in Korea, to sourdough bread, which is thought to have been made originally in Ancient Egypt.

Fermentation is a process of controlled microbial growth, and the goal is to feed and grow the right kinds of bacteria and not the wrong kind. Microorganisms like bacteria break down the fermenting food into simpler compounds, which can enhance its flavour, nutritional value and preserves the food. Fermented products have gained immense popularity worldwide for their health benefits and taste. Unfortunately, just as fibre has been removed from products, many shop-bought 'fermented foods' have been pasteurised to improve shelf life. Some shop-bought sauerkraut products are actually 'vinegar-pickled', which kills the good bacteria so would not be considered a probiotic. You will have to hunt a little bit harder for products that are 'raw' or contain 'live cultures'.

If you want to make your own, it is not as difficult as you might think – see recipes for sauerkraut and kimchi on pages 247 and 249.

## FAT

In medical school I was given quite limited teaching on nutrition. I believe this is true of most medical schools across the country. The lessons we did have followed the now-old-fashioned low-fat dogma – the view that dietary fats are inherently bad for your health. For decades, the theory was believed to be as simple as 'fats make you fat'. However, the idea that fat in the diet leads to fat in the body, which leads to clogging of the arteries, is outdated.

That low-fat dogma triggered an obsession with low-fat, highly processed foods, many of which are in fact worse for you than the full-fat originals. For instance, minimally processed Greek yoghurt contains plenty of fat, however it is likely to be healthier than a highly processed, sugary 'fruit' yoghurt, which may be low in fat but is packed with artificial ingredients to make it palatable. Low-fat yoghurts often contain starchy thickeners and are frequently loaded with extra sugar or sweeteners. For instance, a 2018 study of 136,000 people, across 21 countries, found that those who ate a moderate amount of full-fat dairy products, such as milk, cheese and yoghurt, had a lower risk of heart disease and stroke, when compared to those opting for low-fat alternatives.[9]

When official dietary guidelines were first created in the 1970s, there was a great focus on reducing saturated fats, which had been associated with an increased risk of heart disease. If those saturated fats had been replaced by complex carbohydrates with plenty of fibre (such as beans, lentils, unprocessed oats and sweet potatoes) the outcome may have been different. But in the public's eye, the entire category of 'fat' was tarnished, and we became obsessed with low-fat products. The 'war on fat' had begun: saturated fats were replaced with food items like highly processed, low-fat, high-sugar, carby yoghurts, processed cereals and other so-called low-fat foods.

Cutting down saturated fats, or eating them in moderation, is certainly not an unreasonable idea but, at the time, the health advice recommended filling up on carbohydrates instead. The food industry helpfully stepped in to provide cheap and easy-to-eat refined carbs, such as white bread, cakes, breakfast cereals and biscuits. As these foods are highly processed, many of the original beneficial nutrients were lost as well as the fibre. When they are eaten, they are broken down rapidly by our gut, giving us quick blood sugar spikes and often leaving us feeling unsatisfied and hungry shortly after. The body tries to reduce elevated blood sugar levels by releasing insulin, which redirects that sugar into storage around the body as fat.

Meanwhile, minimally processed dairy, although containing higher levels of fat, also contains lots of helpful nutrients. Removing the fat from yoghurt also removes the fat-soluble vitamins A, D, E and K. A 2019 study found that eating full-fat, fermented foods, such as traditionally made cheese and yoghurt (especially Greek yoghurt), was associated with better metabolic health, and less likelihood of obesity and type 2 diabetes.[10] In moderation they can also be a good source of other nutrients, including protein, calcium, magnesium, iodine and B vitamins.

When eating low-fat products, you have to ask yourself, what are you substituting for the fat?

As well as changes to the guidance on fat, the official nutritional recommendations on eating eggs has changed, too. We used to be told that cholesterol in the diet was linked to cholesterol build-up in the body and, since two eggs contains a whopping 120 per cent of your recommended daily dietary cholesterol allowance, we were told you should limit your egg intake. But that has now been debunked as well. As more evidence has emerged, it appears that dietary cholesterol does not necessarily lead directly to cholesterol in the bloodstream, and governing bodies have removed advice on maximum cholesterol intake. Eaten in moderation, eggs provide an excellent source of protein and nutrients, they keep you full and, for most people, can play an important part of a balanced, healthy diet. It turns out that rather than dietary cholesterol being the problem, the liver produces the vast majority of cholesterol in the body and a diet high in sugar and refined carbs can cause the liver to pump out more cholesterol into the bloodstream, and can also raise levels of inflammation in our blood vessels, which increases the risk of damage and blockages in our arteries.

Many people over the last 40 years switched to low-fat products, and what has happened to obesity levels over that period? They certainly have not gone down – the prevalence of obesity has sky-rocketed.

## HEALTHY FATS

We now know that 'healthy fats' are very good for you and can be your ally in the fight against obesity. There are lots of fats that are incredibly good for your brain and heart, in particular. Do you know which the fattiest organ of the body is? It is the brain, which is 60 per cent fat. One quarter of this fat is a single type of omega-3 called DHA. As a result, omega-3 is vital for healthy brains. It can increase the growth factors in the brain and can even reduce the risk of dementia. Being vital for the health of our brains, various studies have found a strong link between eating fish during pregnancy and a child's IQ.[11] Lack of omega-3 can lead to reduced growth of brain cells.

The best source of omega-3 is found in foods from the sea, particularly oily fish. This is more easily remembered by the acronym SMASH: Sardines, Mackerel, Anchovies, Salmon and Herring. However, other good sources include nuts, seeds, algae and, particularly, seaweed.

Fats have been demonised for decades, yet they are an important part of a balanced diet. As well as the benefits in the fats themselves, adding something like olive oil to a salad or drizzling it onto cooked green vegetables actually makes it easier for our bodies to absorb the nutrients in the vegetables. In fact, there are certain important fat-soluble vitamins that *need* fat for the body to be able to absorb them – vitamins A, D, E and K. When choosing olive oil, aim for extra virgin varieties – they are less likely to be highly processed and so retain more of their natural nutrients.

Seafood was a major component of our Stone Age diets in coastal regions. More than 10,000 years ago, humans survived on hunting, gathering and fishing. Swedish researchers at Lund University looked at the skeletons of 80 individuals who were alive during the Stone Age near a seaside settlement. By performing chemical analyses of the bones, they found that as much as half of their protein intake came from fish. In fact, they found fishing was a common practice not just in seaside regions, but also in freshwater locations, such as settlements nears lakes and rivers.[12]

## Summary

- Whether you are on the jabs or not, it is very important to eat good, real food and to base your eating on the healthy principles of the Mediterranean diet.
- The Mediterranean-style diet is one that consists of plenty of olive oil, whole grains, vegetables, nuts and seeds, as well as moderate amounts of seafood, dairy and poultry.
- Aim to eat plenty of fibre and ideally fermented foods (such as kimchi and sauerkraut) to support your gut microbiome.
- Eat a rainbow of differently coloured fruit and vegetables, in order to maximise your intake of beneficial plant compounds.
- Don't skimp on healthy fats, such as olive oil, avocados, nuts, seeds and oily fish (salmon, sardines, mackerel).

## CHAPTER 10

# HOW TO PROTECT YOUR MUSCLES

As we age, we naturally lose muscle, and there is growing concern that weight loss jabs could accelerate this process and leave people who use them at risk of frailty in older age.

But this doesn't have to be the case. If you eat plenty of protein while you're on the jabs and keep your protein levels up afterwards, and if you incorporate weight-bearing exercises into your routine throughout the whole process, you can preserve and even strengthen your muscles.

One reason for my concern at the potential significance of muscle loss when you're on the weight loss drugs is that the studies that have taken place (funded by the drugs companies) and which show that 25 per cent of the weight loss is lean body mass (of which the main component is muscle) could be deceivingly low. They could be underestimating the level of muscle loss ordinary people might experience. Twenty-five per cent is the proportion of lean body mass loss you might experience through any other form of diet or bariatric surgery, but participants in the SURMOUNT-1 (tirzepatide) and STEP-1 (semaglutide) studies had the benefit of regular counselling on lifestyle changes delivered by health professionals. They were encouraged to eat healthily and exercise for 150 minutes per week. As it states in the SURMOUNT-1 research paper, they advised participants 'to help [them] adhere to healthful, balanced meals, with a deficit of 500 calories per day'.[1] Being a well-funded trial, the participants would have been heavily supervised and supported. Although we do not have the nutritional content of what they ate, it is possible that this could have included plenty of protein to protect their muscles from being broken down in the body's quest for fuel. Inadequate protein intake (very typical on a junk food diet) will accelerate muscle breakdown. My fear is that in the real world where people live more sedentary lives, and without support or lifestyle advice about the importance of eating properly and exercising regularly, it is possible that people on the jabs will lose far more muscle than the studies suggest and, in so doing, will harm their long-term health.

Luckily there are low-cost, cheap and enjoyable options available to reduce muscle loss. The most obvious solutions are eating plenty of protein and exercising, particularly resistance training.

## POWER UP ON PROTEIN

When you think of protein, your mind might flit to the young, fit, gym bunnies with a protein shake in hand, but protein isn't just useful for body builders. It is an essential component of our diets. Every cell in our body uses it. It's needed for growth, the repair of tissues, immune function, the production of enzymes and hormones, as well as for healthy nails and ligaments. Protein is the building block of your muscles, so eating plenty of it helps you to maintain your muscle mass and promotes muscle growth when you exercise. As rapid weight loss causes you to lose muscle as well as fat, one way to help preserve those precious muscles is by eating plenty of good-quality protein.

Unlike other important macronutrients, such as carbohydrates or fat, we are not able to store protein, so we need to have good sources of protein available to eat daily – ideally in every meal. This is even more important if you're taking weight loss drugs. Unless you eat an exemplary diet, when you dramatically reduce your food intake – as people do when taking the medication – your protein intake is likely to dwindle further.

Protein plays an important role in weight maintenance when you come off the jabs, too, because it helps you feel fuller for longer, which means you are less likely to eat the wrong foods and regain the weight you worked so hard to lose. Whether you're on the jabs, coming off the jabs, or you're 'jab curious', it also gets more and more important to incorporate enough protein into your diet as you get older. A big study of people over the age of 50 found that those consuming a daily diet that consisted of at least 1g of protein per kg of body weight (for instance a 70kg woman eating 70g of protein) retained significantly more muscle mass as they lost weight. Not only did they retain *more* muscle, they also lost more fat. It is clear that a higher protein intake when eating a calorie-restricted diet can make a huge difference to how much muscle mass you retain.[2] The authors highlighted the importance of making sure that total protein intake was above the recommended dietary allowance (currently 0.8 g of protein per 1kg of body weight each day) and preferably above 1g of protein per 1kg of body weight.

## Protein for recovery

Recovery from surgical procedures, such as knee or hip replacement, becomes more difficult as we age, and protein is crucial during this healing process in aiding tissue repair and recovery. In the post-op period, you are also more at risk from infection. As we age, our immune systems weaken. Fortunately, getting enough protein helps support the production of immune cells. Adequate protein in the post-op period ultimately speeds up the healing process and reduces the risk of complications. In addition, it can help you preserve your muscle mass, which will, in turn, support your mobility.

## HOW PROTEIN SILENCES HUNGER

Researchers in Australia have identified that our appetite is partly driven by an innate desire for protein. Professor Steve Simpson in Sydney calls this the 'protein leverage hypothesis'. It states that parts of our brain will continue to call for food until our protein needs are met. He believes that this helps to explain why we can still feel hungry after eating a vast amount of food – particularly junk food. If there's not enough protein in that food, our brain will continue to send out 'find more food' messages until it registers that we have eaten the protein we need. He believes this is one reason why we are all eating far more than we need, and gaining weight in ways that were unthinkable back in the 1960s before the proliferation of highly processed food. [3]

Beef-flavoured crisps may have that delicious umami flavour that makes our bodies think we are getting a nice supply of protein, but when that protein doesn't reach our stomach, we are compelled to keep eating to try and get our fill of protein.

Along with fibre, protein helps to reduce the appetite and stabilise blood sugar levels. It takes far fewer calories to get your fill of protein, by eating the likes of chicken, fish, eggs or nuts, compared to the same amount of something like oven-cooked chips.

## HOW TO BOOST YOUR PROTEIN INTAKE

Good, healthy protein comes in the form of meat, fish, eggs, milk and yoghurt, nuts and seeds, beans and pulses, as well as soya products, such as tofu and tempeh (see protein chart on pages 126–7). If you are taking weight loss medication, it is a good idea to aim to make protein the focal point of every meal, because it is a vital tool in your quest to preserve muscle mass.

In an ideal world, you should aim to reach a daily protein score that matches roughly 1g of protein per 1kg of target body weight. So, if you are hoping to reach 70kg, you should try to eat 70g of protein a day. This may be a tricky goal if the appetite-suppressant effect of the jabs means you are eating very little food. But it is important to keep protein levels as high as possible. At every meal, think protein first, then fibre (salad and vegetables), and only add carbohydrates if you are still hungry. It will mean a rethink of how you normally eat breakfast. A small bowl of cornflakes with milk, for instance, will provide 6g of protein, and there's only 3g in a slice of (wholemeal) toast and jam. Check out the breakfast recipes on pages 169–81 for easy ways to increase your protein intake.

When you are coming off the medication, it will be easier to take your protein intake closer to ideal levels. This extra protein in your diet will have the added benefit of keeping you full for longer.

I've heard stories of people who were on the weight loss drugs and knew they needed to increase their protein intake, so pushed their trolley down the supermarket aisle and filled it with anything and everything that had the word 'protein' on the label. This is playing into the hands of Big Food. Some of those proteins may be masquerading as healthy, but are in fact highly processed or contain lots of sugar and starchy additives. If you have the time and the energy, focus on whole food sources of protein as much as you can.

---

## Your protein calculator

The protein content of any food will be less than its overall weight, which takes into account other components (fibre, water, etc.). You'll find protein calculators online, but here are a few useful sources of protein that you can add to your diet:

75g cooked chicken breast – 22.5g
2 slices (80g) roast beef – 26g
2 slices (50g) roast turkey breast – 17g
1 rasher (20g) cooked back bacon – 5g
2 thick slices (40g) ham – 7g

100g steak – 25g

100g minced beef – 20g

100g minced turkey – 27g

75g prawns – 11.5g

45g tuna – 11.5g

1 smoked mackerel fillet (70g) – 15g

2 slices (50g) smoked salmon – 11.5g

100g poached salmon – 24.5g

1 medium egg – 7g

100ml full-fat milk – 3.4g

40g Greek yoghurt – 2g

30g Cheddar – 7.5g

50g feta – 7.5g

30g halloumi – 6g

50g Brie – 10g

100g cottage cheese – 11g

Handful (10g) nuts – 2g

100g cooked beans/chickpeas – 7g

80g cooked edamame beans – 9g

2 tbsp (20g) mixed seeds – 5.4g

100g tofu – 15g

100g cooked lentils – 11g

2 tbsp (50g) hummus – 3.5g

100g cooked quinoa – 6g

## Case study: Simon

Simon is 48 and works as a plasterer. He was training for his black belt in karate but weighed 19 stone and drank up to four fizzy drinks a day. He knew he had to change his diet and lose weight if he was going to pursue his karate ambitions and improve his health. I asked him about his experiences taking Mounjaro.

He says: 'Training for a black belt is incredibly intense and it culminates in a full day of grading. You have a seven-hour day with the grading and the very last half an hour of that day is the fighting. They do that on purpose so that you can retain some level of skill when you're absolutely shattered.

'I was completely committed to my goal. I was four or five stone overweight, blood sugars were high and heading towards, if not already, diabetic. I was exactly the sort of person those jabs were aimed at.

'I've spoken to people who had horrific side effects, if they continued eating and drinking like they did before. I think that's what causes the sickness and diarrhoea. I knew I'd be fine if I ate the right things, so if I had a nice big meal one night, the next night I might have a tin of tuna with some beetroot and no bread, and that's it. The less I ate, the more energy I seemed to have – but that goes back to what I was eating as well. If you eat a McDonalds and a bar of chocolate, you're going to be hungry again in half an hour. If you're having something sensible – a nice ham salad, a bit of tuna, you feel better for longer.

'I was working all day as a plasterer, which is hard work, then training up to four nights a week. So, my physical activity didn't change one bit. In fact, it got more intense as we got closer to the grading. I probably lost some power and some muscle mass – I felt it in the kicks and punches – but it was still an incredibly positive thing.

'If you're not committed, you're more likely to fail. I think a lot of people who have tried these weight loss drugs and haven't changed their lifestyle and their eating habits will find it won't work to the same degree.

'Overall, I dropped from 19 stone 2 pounds to 14 stone 12 pounds which is a massive difference . . . Bouncing around at 19 stone after a 6- or 7-hour day is really difficult, but I found it so much easier to bounce around at 15 stone compared to 19 stone! It was phenomenal, it really was!'

## FLEX THOSE MUSCLES

Eating plenty of protein will help protect your muscles, but exercise is an essential part of the muscle-preserving mix. Multiple studies have shown that you can preserve muscle mass while losing fat on a reduced-calorie diet by incorporating exercise into your day – in particular, resistance training.[4] This is a type of exercise designed to increase the strength of our muscles and it means repeatedly contracting the muscles against a heavy 'resistance' (such as a band or a weight).

Multiple factors act on the muscle to induce growth, including mechanical tension on the muscle, small tears in your muscle fibre, metabolic stress and an increase in certain hormones. The muscle group is overloaded, which signals to the body that muscle needs to grow. After a strength-training workout, the muscle goes into recovery mode and is subsequently rebuilt stronger and thicker than before.

Many may think that these sorts of exercises are just for the young. However, several studies have shown the benefits, not just in those aged 50 to 75 years, but also in older, frailer men and women aged 80 to 100, too![5] Another study compared the strength gains of a group of healthy 65- to 75-year-olds with those of a group of 85-year-olds after 12 weeks in the gym. The younger group had increased muscle mass by 10 per cent with an impressive 38 per cent increase in leg-press strength, but the older group performed even better, increasing muscle mass by 11 per cent and leg strength by 46 per cent.[6] Other studies have shown that resistance training is an effective way to improve muscle strength in the over 75-year-olds and, separately, that it is the most effective way to preserve muscle when following a weight loss diet.[7]

My mother, Clare, spoke to a GP friend of hers who told her about her colleague's adoption of resistance exercises after starting on weight loss drugs. She said: 'He is lifting weights in between patient consultations and it has transformed his health. As a doctor himself, he realised he was at risk of sarcopenia, so he's done his own research.' I believe resistance training should form a very important part of everyone's weight loss journey. If you've never tried strength training before, now is the perfect time to start.

## LET'S GET SWEATY

Depending on your age and mobility, resistance training can take many forms. This could range from 'free weight' training using dumbbells, barbells or kettlebells, to using machines in the gym. Bodyweight exercises, such as press-ups, squats or planks, are another option and can be easily incorporated in the comfort of your home. Others may opt to use resistance bands outdoors or in a group setting. Just pick what suits you best.

Some people find group exercises a great option. We are social animals and it is a great way to meet others and improve our stamina and strength together. It may also provide you with more accountability, and force you out the door to attend a weekly or twice-weekly class. You are less likely to come up with an excuse not to go if it has become embedded in your routine.

The good news for those of us who don't particularly relish the idea of hours in the gym is that studies show that, when it comes to lifting weights, less can sometimes be more. One study showed 30–60 minutes of lifting weights each week offers the greatest reduction in the overall chance of dying from cancer and cardiovascular disease among older adults. Those lifting weights 140 minutes per week or more saw no reduction in mortality compared to those who didn't lift weights at all! These results suggest that many of the health benefits from resistance training can be realised without too much time spent on it. It is reassuring to know that, as we grow older, we do not have to become daily gym rats to see large improvements in our health. A modest amount of strength training may be just as beneficial, if not better.[8]

My dad, Michael, was no lover of exercise. He hated the idea of anything more intense than a brisk walk, and he only did that because he felt he should for health benefits, rather than because he enjoyed it. He was, unfortunately, not someone whose body delivered the flood of feel-good, post-workout chemicals. However, he strategically incorporated exercises, including muscle-strengthening, bodyweight exercises, into his daily routine. That way, he used to say he didn't have to think about it, he just pushed himself through a series of press-ups, squats and several other bodyweight exercises every morning. He was very proud to be able to pump out 35 press-ups at the tender age of 67.

Dad also loved a daily walk in the Buckinghamshire countryside with Mum and their dog, a King Charles Spaniel called Tari. (Honestly, they must have done the same route a few thousand times.) His cardio consisted of cycling up a relatively steep hill back to the house after picking up food from the supermarket. This combination of activities meant that, despite not being a fan of exercise, he was able to incorporate it into his daily life without having to think too much about it.

It's a good idea to pick an exercise routine that is right for you, as he did. Whether that is walking, running, cycling or pumping iron in the gym. There's more than one way to crack a nut. Any small amount of exercise is better than sitting still all day.

## JUST DO IT!

As well as looking after your muscles, pay attention to your heart and lungs, too. Regular exercise can increase our healthspan and improve our chances of leading an independent, active and mobile life in our later years, and for many people it can be an excellent stress buster and mood enhancer, too. Day to day, it can make us feel more alert and improve our concentration span. I interviewed the participants of Professor Roy Taylor's 'Counterbalance Study'[9], as part of my Master of Research in diabetes. I found that those who maintained a good level of activity were successful at keeping the weight off. They told me that even going for a daily walk could lift their mood and motivation. It helped keep them on track with their weight loss journey.

The great thing about exercise? It is never too late to start. One study showed that walking 40 minutes three times a week, in adults aged 55–80 years, increased the size of the hippocampus and improved memory. The hippocampus is the part of your brain responsible for memory and learning, and is one of the first places to be affected by Alzheimer's.[10]

Another study of 20,000 people showed the impact of fitness levels in 'midlife' on developing dementia in later life. It found that the group with the lowest cardiorespiratory fitness were twice as likely to develop dementia as those with higher fitness levels.[11]

---

## No need to overdo it

One study has estimated that 20 minutes of daily 'moderate' aerobic exercise could add 2.2 years to a man's life. Which is worth knowing, because the author of the study calculated that one hour of daily exercise only adds another 0.7 years of life. There are clearly diminishing returns![12]

---

Another big study found that 1–4 hours of vigorous exercise a week (such as running) could reduce your chances of dying, but run for 5 hours and there would be no extra benefit. The authors found the optimal amount of 'moderate exercise' (such as walking) was 5–10 hours a week. Any more than this and any health benefits plateau.[13]

## Case study – Pawel

Pawel is a consultant in emergency medicine in his forties, who works in the northwest. I spoke to him about his experiences on the GLP-1 medication liraglutide. He said: 'When you're really big, you just want to shrink and, to be honest, I don't think you really care whether you lose muscle or fat in the process. But I signed up to The Fast 800 online programme when I was on the jabs and I learned that exercise was an important part of losing weight healthily.

'I was never a sporty person and I thought, "Do I really have to do this?" But when I learned about the health implications of losing my muscles, I started exercising. I'm so grateful that the programme starts you off in a very gradual way – five squats – with no fat shaming.

'I did once sign up for a prescribed lifestyle medicine course but it expected me to go to the gym three times a day. I knew it wasn't for me. The only way I was going to sustain an exercise regime was if I could do it at home with no one watching.

'But with Fast 800 I really got into the exercise videos, and I now go through them every day. I bought a couple of weights and, for the last four years, I've done a half hour routine every morning, I have my gym clothes next to my bed, so I just put them on first thing and get on with it. I feel safe and not judged.

'When you're getting a bit sweaty and breathless, you know it's working.'

## PROTECT YOUR BONES, TOO

Muscles and bones are closely interconnected. Performing resistance exercises, as well as doing any form of impact sports, can help improve bone density, which in turn helps to fend off another major disease of frailty – osteoporosis. This is a condition commonly associated with ageing, which weakens the bones, making them fragile and prone to fracture. Sadly, not everyone who goes into hospital with a hip fracture makes it out again. If we can reduce the risk of fracture in the first place, by staying active and with good nutrition, this could prevent a lot of injuries and deaths.[14]

Osteoporosis can affect men and women of all ages. However, in the first few years after menopause women can lose bone density rapidly, up to 10 per cent within the first 5 years, due to a drop in oestrogen. This can really increase your risk of osteoporosis. You may not know you suffer from this 'silent disease' until you either fracture a bone or undergo a scan.

You can protect yourself against osteoporosis by eating a good diet with plenty of calcium, taking part in regular strength training, doing impact exercise (for example tennis, jogging or dancing) and reducing your consumption of alcohol, caffeine or smoking.

## Summary

- Exercising, including strength training, and increasing your protein intake will help to offset muscle loss.
- Aim for at least 2 days per week of muscle strength training – at least 30–60 minutes (over the week). You are never too old to start.
- Aim for 75 minutes of vigorous intensity exercise or 150 minutes of moderate intensity aerobic activity each week.
- Choose a form of exercise that you enjoy and always build it into your daily routine so it happens without you having to make a decision.

# CHAPTER 11

# THE PLAN

Having read the previous chapters, you will have an understanding of how the weight loss medications work, and how important it is to focus on eating a healthy diet and exercising regularly to ensure the weight stays off long-term. Now it's time to put it all into practice.

This plan should help you find a healthy and sustainable route to rapid weight loss. It also incorporates a clever routine for easing you back into normal life once you start reducing your drug dose, with crucial advice for helping you maintain your new healthy weight, should you choose that route.

When we sat down as a family to think about the best way to support a healthy diet and lifestyle when someone is on the medication and afterwards, we realised a solution was staring us in the face: The Fast 800 programme. This is the diet dad pioneered and was so passionate about.

Dad had been closely following the development of the weight loss drugs. He always promoted a 'diet and lifestyle first' approach, yet he could see how the GLP-1 medications had the potential to help huge numbers of people. Here are some of his thoughts on the subject:

'Historically, I have been very sceptical about weight loss potions and pills because, frankly, they come with a long history of quackery and most of them have either been ineffective, or they have some really nasty side effects. But what makes these GLP-1 drugs so different is they have been shown in randomised controlled trials to be both safe and effective. Although, they are not without side effects. Having said that, compared to anything we've seen before, they really are quite remarkable.

'Of course, there has also been lots of evidence that when you stop taking the drug, hunger returns and the weight goes back on. Some people report feeling even hungrier – a sort of rebound reaction. So, unless you have made lifestyle changes, you will start to regain that lost weight and quite a lot of that weight is going to be fat. You risk ending up in a slightly worse position than you were when you started.

'But I don't see these new GLP-1 drugs as an alternative to The Fast 800. I think they're actually complementary.

'Using these drugs can be effective at helping you lose weight in the short term. But if you want to keep the weight off long term, you're going to need to learn how to eat more healthily, how to exercise to maintain your muscle mass, and how to use stress reduction techniques to help you when you are feeling under pressure. Because unless you have that backup system going, the danger is that, in the long term, you will just put the weight back on again.

'If it's suitable for you, then combining one of these drugs with The Fast 800 programme might offer the best of both worlds. The drugs will help suppress your appetite, but you really do need some sort of programme in order to change your habits, learn better ways of eating and get enough protein and fibre in your diet.

'Losing weight might be an excellent goal, but we should all be working towards a lifestyle that continues to support better health long term. When you combine GLP-1s with The Fast 800 programme, you learn how to eat and live well, and you'll have all the tools you need to maintain your weight.'

Dad could see that these drugs could be a useful tool but should not replace the toolbox altogether. So, we have adapted the three-stage Fast 800 plan to pull everything together and to make sure you really do get the best of both worlds.

It is important to consider that there are already effective and rapid, drug-free routes to long-term weight loss (with Professor Roy Taylor from Newcastle leading the charge with his latest research – see page 150). Many thousands of people now follow The Fast 800 programme. Recent validated data looking at 23,745 people who used The Fast 800 plan (without the weight loss medications), found there was an average weight loss of 7.3kg for those living with obesity after only 12 weeks, as well as showing a significant reduction in blood sugars for those with diabetes and prediabetes.

Rapid weight loss has had an unfair rap for decades. However, the amount of weight you lose in the first few weeks of a diet is a predictor of how much you keep off in the long run. If approached correctly, those with excess weight can see phenomenal results, and a rapid improvement in metabolic health. Studies clearly show that a low-calorie diet can reverse type 2 diabetes and shed a vast amount of fat directly from your liver.

Over the past decade, rapid weight loss and intermittent fasting have gained significant popularity. Resources like the books *The Fast 800* and *The Fast 800 Keto Recipe Book*, along with programmes, such as The Fast 800 programme, provide valuable information and support. You can explore more at www.thefast800.com.

## The diamond trial

In 2019, my mum was one of the authors of a small study led by Professor Susan Jebb from the Nuffield Department of Primary Care Health Sciences in Oxford. This was a randomised control trial comparing a regimen where participants consumed 800–1000 calories per day, following a lowish-carb, Mediterranean-style diet (similar to The Fast 800), using real food, to participants following the standard UK healthy- and balanced-eating guidelines.

Although it was a small trial in overweight diabetics, the results were very encouraging. Participants showed significant weight loss over three months: 9.5kg, compared to only 2.5kg in the control group. They also demonstrated an impressive drop in average blood sugar of 16.3mmol/mol, compared to 0.7mmol/mol in the control. The trial showed that extremely impressive results could be achieved through diet alone. This was delivered in primary care by nurses over five extended consultations. This is now being followed up as a much larger study.[1]

## But first, STOP and think –
## are weight loss drugs right for you?

Just because your friend, neighbour, work colleague or partner is using weight loss injections, it doesn't mean this route is healthy or appropriate for you. If you have any doubts about whether it is the right course for you, I urge you to arrange a face-to-face consultation with a qualified health professional for an assessment. Don't rush into trying to get hold of these drugs without properly thinking through what you're doing.

Ask yourself:

- Am I prepared for the ongoing cost? (These drugs are not a quick fix, and unless you change your diet and lifestyle you might have to consider taking them for a prolonged period.)
- Am I prepared for the possible side effects, such as nausea and constipation, vomiting and diarrhoea?
- Am I prepared to risk losing some enjoyment in food?
- Am I prepared to put a drug in my body that hasn't had long-term safety studies at the doses currently being taken?
- Is this drug right for me? (As of 2024, caution is recommended for anyone with a history of pancreatitis, gall stones or thyroid cancer, and it is not currently recommended for anyone with a BMI under 27, or anyone pregnant or breastfeeding. This is a non-exhaustive list – look at the up-to-date drug manufacturers' instructions for a complete list.)
- How will I set myself up for success when coming off the weight loss medications?
- Could I achieve the same results without resorting to medication?

If you are still convinced that the weight loss medication may help you lose weight, then just make one solid commitment for your health: promise you will combine the medication with significant improvements to your diet and lifestyle.

It would also be wise to pair the drugs with a suitable book, such as *The Fast 800 Keto Recipe Book*, and/or with a good-quality support programme, such as The Fast 800 Programme (www.thefast800.com). The advice and recipes are designed to provide adequate protein, fibre and nutrients to support your needs, while calorie restricting. You can also benefit from The Fast 800 tailored exercises to preserve your muscles, access to a supportive community, apply simple behavioural changes, mindfulness and more.

### Exclusions and cautions for rapid weight loss

Cautions: Rapid weight loss does not suit everyone. If you have a significant underlying medical condition, for example type 2 diabetes, are on insulin or other medication; if you have high blood pressure, moderate or severe retinopathy, epilepsy, gallstones, cardiac issues, thyroid disorders, kidney disease, severe liver disease; or if you are immune compromised, pregnant or breast-feeding, please talk to your doctor before going on this diet.

Exclusions: This diet is not suitable for teenagers, people with a history of an eating disorder or a psychiatric illness, or if you are unwell, underweight or doing endurance exercise.

See more at: www.thefast800.com/frequently-asked-questions/

## THREE-STAGE PLAN
### Stage 1: Rapid weight loss

When you reach the right dose of the medications, your appetite will be suppressed and you will want to eat much less than you used to. Some people relish the thought of skipping meals and going through the whole day eating virtually nothing, but it is very important to maximise your nutritional intake. Think of this stage as a great opportunity to retrain your eating habits and build your appreciation of healthy foods.

With a reduced appetite, you are likely to reduce your food intake without effort. Generally, we would suggest 800–1000 calories per day during the rapid weight loss phase. However, if you are using the weight loss drugs, your appetite may be significantly suppressed, your weight may be flying off and counting calories may not be necessary. You might even notice a significant reduction in your alcohol intake, too.

The jabs are likely to make you feel queasy at the thought of deep-fried foods, so listen to those messages and don't fall into the trap of wasting your now tiny appetite on junk that will not fuel your body effectively. People who experience side effects, such as vomiting and diarrhoea, often say this happens when they eat too much unhealthy food (or when they are on too high a dose).

Another key message here is to reduce your intake of starchy carbohydrates, such as white bread, white rice and white pasta, as they rapidly break down into sugars in the blood. Make a concerted effort to avoid UPFs, which often contain large quantities of refined carbs and sugars. Instead, base your eating on a lowish carbohydrate, Mediterranean-style diet, rich in olive oil, seeds, fruit, eggs, vegetables, pulses and fish, alongside moderate amounts of meat and dairy products. This has been shown to promote weight loss, maintain muscle mass and keep you properly nourished.

The recipes in this book will provide plenty of inspiration.

### Prioritise two main nutrients

Protein: If you don't eat enough protein (at least 60g per day) when you are on weight loss medications, your body will scavenge protein from your muscles, resulting in loss of lean muscle mass (see Chapter 10: How to Protect Your Muscles). So, it is important to make protein, such as fish, chicken, cheese, eggs, nuts or tofu, a significant part of each meal.

Fibre: Aim for 30g of dietary fibre every day to keep your gut microbiome happy and healthy. Do this by eating as many vegetables, beans, nuts and seeds as you can, and add some wholegrains, too. Fibre is crucial for maintaining a functioning digestive tract, which will mitigate any unwanted side effects, such as constipation or diarrhoea. And you will be feeding a healthy gut microbiome in the process, which will benefit your health and mood.

### Drink plenty of water

As you burn fat, your body naturally loses fluid, particularly in the early days, so keep yourself well hydrated by adding an extra 1–1.5 litres of water a day, or more if it's hot or you are exercising. Dehydration can leave to you feeling drained and irritable, as well as causing headaches and exacerbating constipation. These are powerful drugs and some people have even ended up in hospital with significant dehydration. To check hydration, pay attention when you pass urine – your wee should be the colour of lemonade and you should be passing a good volume six to eight times a day.

Drink water and herbal teas, and jazz things up by adding a slice of orange, lemon, cucumber or perhaps some strawberries or mint to your water. Cold sparkling water can be refreshing, too.

*Be active*

Keeping active throughout this and every stage of the plan is very important. To avoid losing muscle (which can be hard to regain), you need to incorporate some kind of strength training into your weekly routine. Don't wait until you've lost weight – this needs to start right now! (Again, see Chapter 10: How to Protect Your Muscles.) Those following The Fast 800 programme have easy access to online guided videos that help to improve their strength and fitness. Or you could join an exercise class with other people. This is a social way to do it and you can learn good techniques, too. Gyms normally have classes for a range of abilities. Alternatively, you could buy a few dumbbells or just use your own body weight and exercise from the comfort of your own home.

## Stage 2: Coming off the jabs

Congratulations, you've nearly reached your target and you'll be thinking about reducing your injection dosage. This is a significant point in your weight loss journey. But please don't just stop taking the drugs and hope for the best. It is important for you to check in with your health professional at this stage, so they can help you create a plan for tapering off or stopping the medication, and they may also assess your metabolic health, blood pressure and any other potential risk areas, which are likely to be considerably improved.

As you reduce your dose of the medication, you may notice a return of food noise. But don't fall into the trap of old habits. The online community group provided via The Fast 800 programme is an added dose of support from likeminded individuals who are also working their way through food noise and other challenges. Collaboration with others is key to sustained success. If you redouble your focus on a lowish carbohydrate, Mediterranean-style diet, packed with protein and healthy fats and plenty of vegetables, you shouldn't be tormented by cravings.

### Eat good food

By now, the lowish carbohydrate, Mediterranean-style diet you've been sticking to throughout the rapid weight loss phase should be starting to feel familiar. You will understand the importance of protein and fibre in every meal, and you will have enjoyed experimenting with some of the recipes in this book.

As your appetite returns, you should make sure you are hitting your protein and fibre targets (page 144). As long as you stick to the healthy-eating guidelines I have laid out, you can afford to eat larger portions to satisfy that increased hunger. If you base your meals on good proteins, fibre and healthy fats, you will feel fuller for longer and you are likely to feel better in your mood, too, all of which will help you keep away from unhealthy, processed junk foods.

*Try fasting – 3:4, 5:2 or even 6:1*

Without the medication to dampen your appetite, you may feel hungrier on some days than others. It can help to incorporate a bit of intermittent fasting – allocating two or three days each week to restricting your calorie intake or eating smaller portions (keeping calories to 800–1000 per day), then eating larger portions on the other days. This is low enough to mimic the effects of fasting, which aids weight loss, but without you having to feel too hungry.

Not only is having fasting days like this a very effective fat-burning tool, but it also provides a range of other health benefits. When your body thinks you are fasting, it switches from 'growth mode' to 'repair mode'. Fasting can reduce inflammation, which improves heart and brain health and prompts cellular repair. It can even reduce the risk of certain cancers. When your body switches into repair mode, a clean-up operation begins – the body removes damaged cells and forms healthier ones – a process called autophagy.

Follow a pattern that suits you – from the more intense 3:4 pattern (four days 'fasting' each week), to the 5:2, or 6:1 (if you are approaching your weight loss goals). Some people find it easier to fast during the week and take a more relaxed approach on the weekends. Fasting has been shown to be an effective way to maintain weight loss and it can even keep the numbers on the scales creeping slowly downwards. It can work just as effectively, whether you are still on a low dose of the weight loss drugs or if you've stopped taking them.

## Weigh yourself regularly

Studies show that keeping a close eye on your weight makes it much easier to nip small weight gains in the bud, rather than having to tackle a great big tranche of weight loss again. Throw in some extra 'fast' days if you do notice your weight creeping up.

## Time Restricted Eating (TRE)

Another intermittent fasting trick you might like to incorporate at this stage is 'time restricted eating' (TRE), which extends your overnight fast by a few hours to harness all the lovely benefits of fasting (and helps keep your weight in check). Pick a pattern that suits you – it might be as simple as eating a slightly late breakfast and having an early evening meal, or skipping breakfast entirely and just eating two meals a day. To begin with, you could try a 12:12 pattern (12 hour overnight fast). If you feel this is easy and want to be more ambitious, you could extend it to 14:10 (14 hour overnight fast).

Whatever method you use, just ensure you eat a healthy Mediterranean diet. Try and keep the processed junk foods to a minimum and avoid keeping them in your cupboards at home. During this phase, the weight loss is likely to be less rapid, but you will be building good nutritional habits to carry you into the future.

## Exercise

Exercise should be a habitual part of your life now, and you should be getting into a rhythm of regular sessions of strength training to keep those muscles strong. Muscle really matters: it is metabolically active and requires more energy to maintain than fatty tissue. People with greater muscle mass burn more calories even when they are not exercising. Muscle keeps us young and fit, and it reduces the risk of type 2 diabetes and future frailty. For maximum benefit, combine strength training with aerobic exercise.[2]

---

## HICT

One great way of combing cardio and strength training is High Intensity Circuit Training (HICT). Search '7-minute workout' online for free versions. Or you can access workouts via The Fast 800. HICT is an easy way to get into resistance exercises and it kills two birds with one stone: cardio and strength together. The great thing about HICT is that it is a full body workout that only requires a chair and takes just 7 minutes to complete. It is especially helpful if your focus is to improve your functional muscles as you age, but it will get you in better shape, too.

---

*Nail your motivation*

Weight loss is made so much easier if you've got weight loss drugs silencing the food noise and the numbers are tumbling on the scales week by week, but when you stop taking the drugs, the food noise might try to tempt you back into your previously unhelpful, and probably unhealthy, patterns of eating.

At this stage you'll need to hang on to whatever motivated you to lose weight in the first place – to feel more confident or more energised? To play with your children or your grandchildren without rapidly getting out of breath? To reverse diabetes? To put off a knee replacement? Whatever your reason, write it down now and display it somewhere prominent to remind you when your willpower wavers.

As part of my medical studies, I completed a Master of Research in diabetes with Professor Roy Taylor, who worked closely with my dad, Michael, over the years. One of my tasks was following up with the participants from Professor Taylor's 'Counterbalance Study', which had showed for the first time that rapid weight loss could reverse type 2 diabetes.[3] My job was to interview the participants several years after the study had been completed, and to identify any factors that might have aided or hindered their weight loss maintenance.

I discovered that for some people a disruptive life event (fracturing a leg, changing jobs, having to work away from home) could lead them to 'falling off the wagon'. They rapidly found themselves descending into a vicious cycle, where the healthy-eating habits that had helped them lose weight went right out of the window.

Some studies show healthy mental wellbeing to be crucial to maintaining weight loss.[4] Other research investigating relapse from various addictions[5] shows there can be a lot of guilt and stigma associated with relapse, and that this shame can prompt binge eating. However, to sustain healthy habits and keep the weight maintenance on track, it is very important to remove the stigma from these episodes, and to allow people to realise that these are a normal part of the weight loss journey.[6]

After working with Professor Taylor, I identified a 'motivational cycle' when weight was lost or kept off. Factors that seemed to really help keep people on the straight and narrow included having a sense of improved physical wellbeing and mood, managing effective goal setting, doing regular exercise, and having a supportive partner. Together, these seem to help people hang on to the motivation to eat a better diet and so maintain weight loss.

## Stage 3: Long-term success

Hopefully, by this stage, you have reached your weight loss goal and improved your metabolic health.

You may decide to stop the GLP-1 medications at this point. I believe coming off or at least reducing the medication should be a goal for most people. If your weight does rebound substantially when you stop taking the GLP-1s and you are really struggling, it is not unreasonable to ask your health-care provider about restarting the medications at a low dose, at least until you feel you have things more under control.

By now, your Mediterranean-style diet should be the norm and you will be familiar with eating plenty of protein, healthy fats, fibre and coloured fruit and vegetables. Exercise and strength training should continue to be a non-negotiable part of your healthy regime.

Here's a summary of what foods to eat:

1. Avoid processed junk foods – high in calories, low in nutrition.
2. Eat plenty of protein – hold onto that precious muscle.
3. Eat plenty of fibre – helps regulate your bowels, but also great for your gut microbiome and thus your body and brain.

4. Eat healthy fats, such as oily fish, nuts, seeds, avocados and olive oil – good for the brain and the heart, and they keep you feeling full.

5. Enjoy complex carbohydrates, such as wholegrains, beans and legumes – a good source of fibre.

6. Eat a rainbow of colourful fruit and vegetables – packed with a variety of phytonutrients, vitamins and minerals.

This maintenance phase can be dynamic. Continue to weigh yourself regularly and you can always bring back in a few fasting days if you feel the weight starting to creep up again.

Whether or not you dip in and out of medication in the future, it is incredibly important to eat nutritious, filling food, and to maintain a good amount of activity. Resistance training now will help to ensure that, if you do regain a little of the lost weight, it will be healthy, life-affirming muscle and not fat. Prioritising sleep and stress management will also help you stay on track.

---

### 12 tips for success

1. Clear your kitchen cupboards of temptation. Empty them of processed junk foods – willpower is overrated. It will be far harder to succumb to temptation and reach for your favourite sugary and salty snack if they are not there!

2. Weigh yourself regularly. Studies show that doing so can help you keep on track.

3. Bring your partner or a friend on board. Having someone who is supporting you on your weight loss and healthy-eating journey can make it easier. It can provide accountability too.

4. Build in good habits. Cycle to work, take the stairs not the lift, do resistance exercises first thing in the morning, and leave your exercise clothes next to your bed.

5. Swap to healthy snacks (see recipes on pages 231–44). If you love a good snack, dump the processed junk and enjoy moderate portions of nuts, seeds, Greek yoghurt, cheese, or veg sticks and hummus. Swap crisps for nuts, milk chocolate for dark, and biscuits for fruit.

6. Eat whole foods most of the time.

7. Plan your meals ahead. Set aside time on a Sunday evening to plan meals for the week. Pick out the recipes and ingredients when you've got time to think about what you need. Many of the meals can also be cooked in batches and set aside in the fridge or freezer for a day when you are more squeezed for time.

8. Remind yourself of your motivation. A health concern, such as trying to reverse type 2 diabetes, staying off blood pressure pills, avoidance of knee surgery, or minimising back pain, can provide stronger and more effective motivation than simply 'I want to look slimmer'. Healthspan can be big a motivation, too. Few people

would say they want to live longer if their quality of life is poor due to significant weight-related health problems. Losing excess weight can also help with better sleep, more energy, less joint pain, better mobility and enhanced mood – a greater zest for life.

9. Don't punish yourself for an overindulgence. If you slip up, don't throw in the towel. Be kind yourself and don't allow guilt to creep in. A 2014 study found that those participants who associated 'guilt' with eating a forbidden food item, such as a chocolate cake, had poorer control over what they ate and were less likely to maintain their weight loss.[7]

10. Celebrate how much fitter and healthier you feel than you did before. A Mediterranean-style diet can lift your mood and, paired with exercise, it can help create a virtuous cycle of feeling good, which makes it easier to stick to eating well.

11. Have a good night's sleep. Poor diet can lead to bad sleep and obesity-related health problems, such as sleep apnoea, and lack of sleep can lead to overeating and poor food choices. A recent Danish study showed that, after a period of 13kg weight loss, the participants who slept badly were more likely to regain the weight.[8] Poor sleep can lead to increased appetite, and it can also lead to higher levels of the stress hormone cortisol, which can increase your blood sugar levels. Luckily there is evidence that a better diet (higher protein, high fibre) can enhance your sleep quality.

12. Eat slowly. Chew your food, enjoy it, eat mindfully . . . This is easier done with whole foods, which require more mastication.

Many processed junk foods will quite literally melt in your mouth, and before you know it you've inhaled the whole pack.

## Summary

- Don't rush into any decision to take weight loss medication. A non-medicated route (such as The Fast 800) may be effective for you.
- Stage 1: Rapid weight loss. When you are taking the weight loss jabs, avoid junk food and eat a Mediterranean-style diet of whole foods, prioritising protein (at least 60g per day) and fibre (30g vegetables, beans, lentils, seeds and wholegrains). Drink plenty of water and start a resistance-training exercise programme.
- Stage 2: Coming off the jabs. Seek professional advice about coming off the medication and gradually lowering your dose. Stick with the Mediterranean-style diet, prioritising protein and fibre, and ensuring protein intake of at least 1g per 1kg of body weight. Consider adding intermittent fasting (sticking to 800–1000 calories on certain days of the week, and eating normally on the other days) and consider Time Restricted Eating (restricting your eating window to 8–12 hours) to keep weight loss on track. Keep exercising.
- Stage 3: Long-term success. Continue eating a healthy Mediterranean-style diet, weighing yourself regularly, and throwing in a few fasting days if the weight creeps back on. Keep up with the exercise.

# CONCLUSION

We are standing on the precipice of a new era in obesity treatment. These new weight loss medications represent a huge breakthrough, but it is clear they also throw up significant challenges.

For the first time in history, we have medications that can lead to major weight loss, and for those millions of people who have struggled with their weight, often for many decades, these drugs hold a significance that cannot be underestimated.

But the new weight loss drugs shine a rather shady light on the complex issues that got us here in the first place. Unless we take steps to diminish the power of Big Food to deliver highly processed, calorie-dense yet nutritionally depleted junk food, which has been cynically designed to be consumed in excess, we will only be switching one set of health challenges for another.

The weight loss drugs could help bring the obesity epidemic under control, which could potentially save the NHS the billions of pounds it currently spends on dealing with obesity-related diseases. Recent estimates suggest that unhealthy eating costs the country £268 billion per year in the UK, in terms of productivity, health and care costs.[1]

But these drugs could herald serious health problems in the future. Unless the people who are taking them take steps to switch to eating real, nutritious food, and work hard to maintain their muscle mass as their weight drops away, they could become increasingly malnourished and frail.

## FREELY AVAILABLE ON THE NHS?

Although these drugs may not fix healthy eating (much as we'd like them to), they could certainly play a role in helping solve the obesity crisis. The government is talking about possibly rolling out the weight loss drugs on the NHS over the next few years but cost is a restrictive factor.

The problem is that 3.4 million people qualify under the current NICE guidelines for NHS drug support, but the already squeezed NHS simply does not have the capacity or funding to roll the drugs out safely, while also providing a more holistic approach and support.

Those who do receive the medications for weight loss can be prescribed the drugs for a maximum of two years. This has the potential to be a sensible solution, given that the medication's long-term risks are still being studied. However, given that the average person puts back on most of the weight they lost after one year off the GLP-1s, giving the medication for just two years could be problematic.

Nevertheless, the NHS has declared it intends to provide Mounjaro (tirzepatide) to a quarter of a million people over the next three years.[2] A five-year NHS trial is currently underway in Manchester, looking at how best to implement the medications. The aim of the trial is to use the weight loss medications to help prevent obesity-related disease and ease the strain on the NHS. The UK government has also indicated its goal to encourage people who have struggled to work due to obesity-related illnesses to get back into work.

## FOCUS ON DIET

For a roll out of the weight loss medications to be successful, a greater focus on dietary advice will be key. This could take the form of more education in up-to-date lifestyle advice for patient-facing staff.

You certainly can't argue with the vital impact a healthy diet has on our health, but there is still a woeful lack of teaching about lifestyle and diet to healthcare workers. Reassuringly, NICE has recommended the implementation of 'a range of community-based services and digital technologies' to assist the provision of the weight loss medications.[3]

I share the view of many medics that a digital service of some form or other, coupled with support from a health practitioner, is almost essential to provide the extra resources and advice desperately required to support those taking the weight loss medications. Dietary and lifestyle advice, support and guidance is needed now more than ever.

## THE HAVES AND THE HAVE-NOTS

In the short term, these drugs are only really available to those who can afford to pay for them. Certainly, most people using them in the UK are paying privately – anything from £150 to £300 per month. As things stand, it is a case of the haves and have-nots; those who can afford the medications are able to acquire it, primarily through online pharmacies; those who cannot afford them, some of whom could derive significant benefits, are struggling to get access.

The good news is that both availability and price of the weight loss medications should keep coming down, as new drugs make it to the market and competition among the drug companies heats up. The drugs will come off patent in the early 2030s (they will become generic, like paracetamol and ibuprofen), which means you will be able to buy much cheaper versions and see a five- or even tenfold drop in price. When this happens, I am hopeful that the NHS can find the right strategy to allow people to use these medications in a safe and structured way.

## EXCITING TIMES

There's no doubt GLP-1s are here to stay and I believe we will see their impact grow more and more as we move towards the end of the decade. The impact of relatively easy weight loss will affect individuals and society, for better or for worse, in ways we may not yet know.

We are living in exciting times for the world of weight loss. The way these powerful drugs muffle the siren call of addictive processed junk foods provides us with a unique opportunity to change the way we eat and live.

My father, Michael, believed in empowering people with the knowledge and practical tools to take control of their own health. My hope is that this book might provide, in his memory, a blueprint that could equip as many people as possible with the knowledge they need to make informed decisions, and use these fascinating new weight loss drugs safely.

# Q&A

## WHAT SIDE EFFECTS SHOULD I TAKE SERIOUSLY?

Common side effects include nausea, diarrhoea, constipation, occasional vomiting and mild headaches. Talk to your GP (and always explain you are taking weight loss jabs) if you are concerned. But anyone with severe abdominal pain or persistent vomiting should seek immediate medical help. If you have signs of an allergic reaction, such as swelling, a rash or shortness of breath, seek urgent medical attention.

## IF I DON'T FEEL HUNGRY, CAN I SKIP MEALS OR JUST EAT SNACKS?

Eating real whole foods is essential, as is focusing on protein and fibre, especially while taking the GLP-1 medications. It will help you avoid muscle loss and even malnutrition. You will feel much better, too. At all costs, you want to avoid being both underfed and undernourished!

## WHAT IF I CAN'T OR DON'T HAVE TIME TO COOK?

Time and convenience is, of course, a big part of the appeal of processed junk foods, but please don't succumb! The recipes in this book are delicious and straightforward, with few ingredients. You can save time by cooking in batches and freezing meals, so you have leftovers easily to hand.

## WHAT IF I LOVE SNACKING?

Try and swap those sweet or salty processed foods with healthy and nutritious alternatives, such as nuts, some fruit, a few slices of cheese, or carrot sticks with hummus.

## CAN I FOLLOW THIS PLAN
## IF I AM VEGETARIAN OR VEGAN?

There are plenty of vegetarian and pescatarian recipes in this book. The diet is more difficult for vegans, as it can be harder to get enough protein. Double your focus on good-quality foods like tofu, tempeh, nuts, edamame beans, lentils, beans, nutritional yeast and seitan. See pages 126–7 for protein top-up suggestions. It might help to add vegan protein powder.

## HOW DO I DEAL WITH CONSTIPATION?

Eat fibrous vegetables with every meal to ensure you have lots of fibre on board and drink plenty of water (an extra 1–1.5 litres is needed when losing weight, and more if it's hot or you are exercising). If you suffer from vomiting or diarrhoea, as a side effect of taking the medication, you could be at greater risk of dehydration. Drinking plenty of fluids will help reduce constipation and may improve your energy, too.

## HOW CAN I AVOID DEHYDRATION?

When you lose weight rapidly, you release water as you burn fat. So, it is important to add an extra 1–1.5 litres of fluid each day, and more if it is hot or you are exercising. One of the most common side effects of losing weight, particularly at first, is dehydration. This can leave you feeling drained, with a headache and fatigue. Another common impact of getting dehydrated is that it makes you constipated –a frequent side effect of the drug.

So it's important to be on top of your hydration. A good guide to avoid dehydration is to check that your urine is the colour of lemonade and that you are passing 6 to 8 good volumes of urine a day.

This is one of the reasons that many of the recipes include plenty of fibre in the form of beans, lentils, wholegrains, fruit and vegetables.

Many people are happy to drink water, carry a bottle or keep a cold jug in the fridge. Make herbal teas and drink them hot or cold.

## IF I HAVE SIGNIFICANT SYMPTOMS – VOMITING, DIARRHOEA, CONSTIPATION – SHOULD I INCREASE THE DOSE OF THE GLP-1S?

My inclination would be to say absolutely not! You should consider seeking medical advice. Unfortunately, many online pharmacies appear to be encouraging users to increase their doses, almost no matter what. Be careful.

## WHICH DRUG IS WHICH?

Semaglutide (Ozempic, Wegovy)

Tirzepatide (Mounjaro, Zepbound)

Retatrutide (still in clinical trials)

Liraglutide (Saxendra)

## SHOULD I TELL MY DOCTOR
## I AM TAKING THE GLP-1 MEDICATIONS?

Yes, absolutely. A responsible online pharmacist should inform your GP, but you cannot assume this has happened.

## ISN'T IT BAD TO LOSE WEIGHT REALLY FAST?

Not necessarily. For people who are living with obesity, rapid weight loss can be beneficial and the dangers have been debunked. In one study, those who achieved faster initial weight loss were more than five times more likely to have kept the weight off, and lost more than 10 per cent of their body weight over the longer term (at the 18 months mark).[1] But, as with any diet, it is always wise to check with a health professional first, not least for the support they might be able to give.

## CAN I USE MEAL REPLACEMENT SHAKES?

Aim to focus on eating whole foods as much as possible. However, a good-quality meal replacement shake can be useful if taken occasionally when you don't have time to prepare a nutritious meal. My dad, Michael, sometimes used low-sugar, high-protein and high-fibre shakes when he was away from home filming as an alternative to unhealthy snacks or canteen food.

As a junior doctor, I have worked night shifts in the NHS and in Australia, and I found them really challenging. My motivation to eat a nicely prepared meal on these shifts was pretty low – I just wanted accessible, hyperpalatable, addictive sweet and salty snacks. That impetus is one reason why shift work, and night shifts in particular, can take years off your life. In circumstances like these, having something simple, like a nutritional shake (as long as it is higher in protein and fibre, low in sugar, and contains vitamins and minerals), could provide a reasonable alternative to grabbing a pastry or pasty.

Professor Roy Taylor has conducted several studies to show that weight loss and remission from type 2 diabetes is possible using meal replacement soups and shakes with additional vegetables. For research purposes, using nutritionally complete soups and shakes allows the study methods to be standardised more easily and can allow better control of the calories the participants are taking. The participants who completed the study lost an average of 16kg (14.4 per cent of their body weight) and 32 per cent of the participants saw remission of their type 2 diabetes. The study was performed without the assistance of weight loss drugs. The results were so impressive that the NHS is now rolling out the Type 2 Diabetes Path to Remission Programme, in which patients are provided nutritionally complete shakes, soups and bars, on the back of this research.[2]

# 7-DAY MEAL PLAN

**Day 1**
**Mango and lime chia pots** (page 169)
**Quick spinach and pea soup** (pages 181–2)
**Roasted salmon and courgettes with anchovy chilli butter**
(pages 201–2)

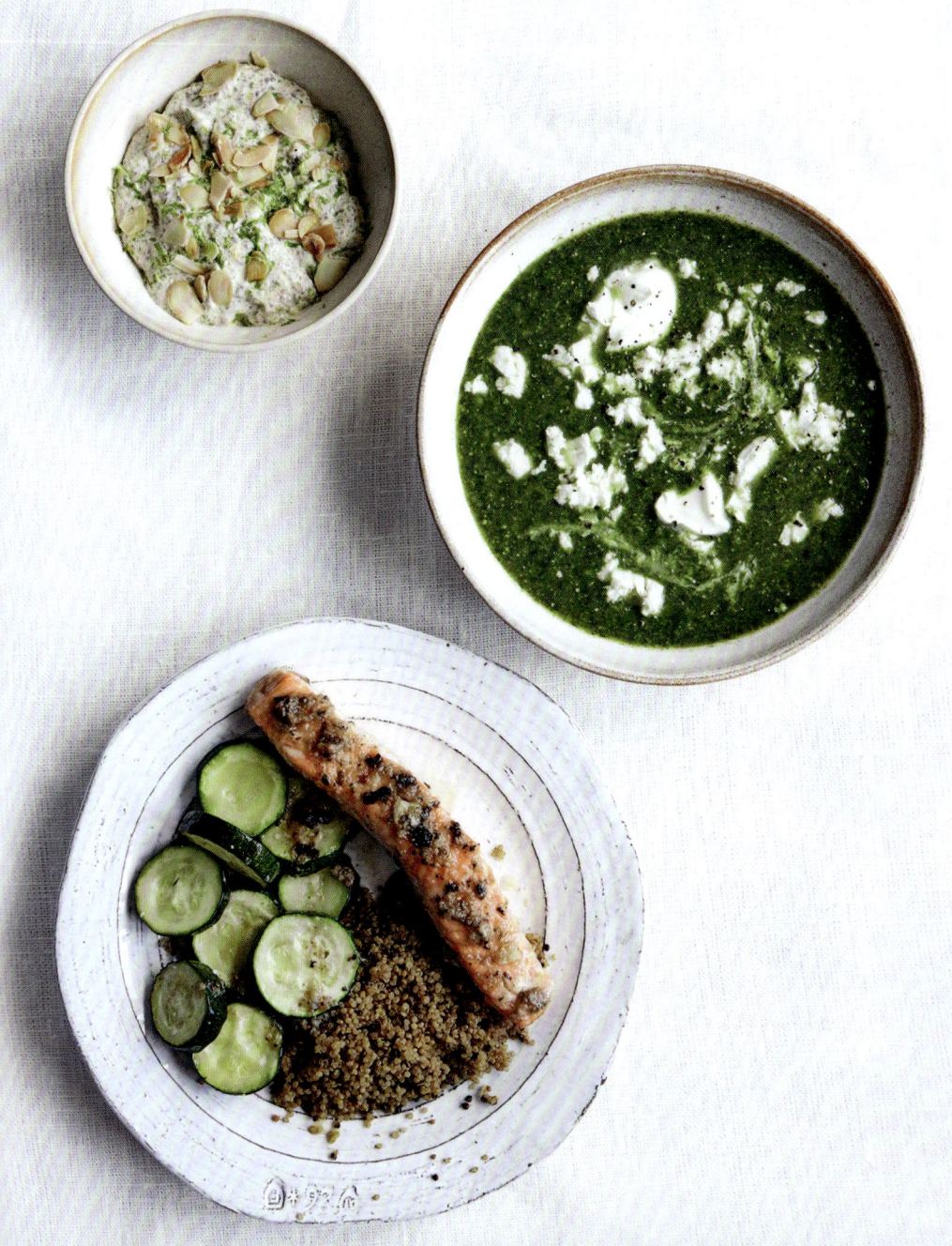

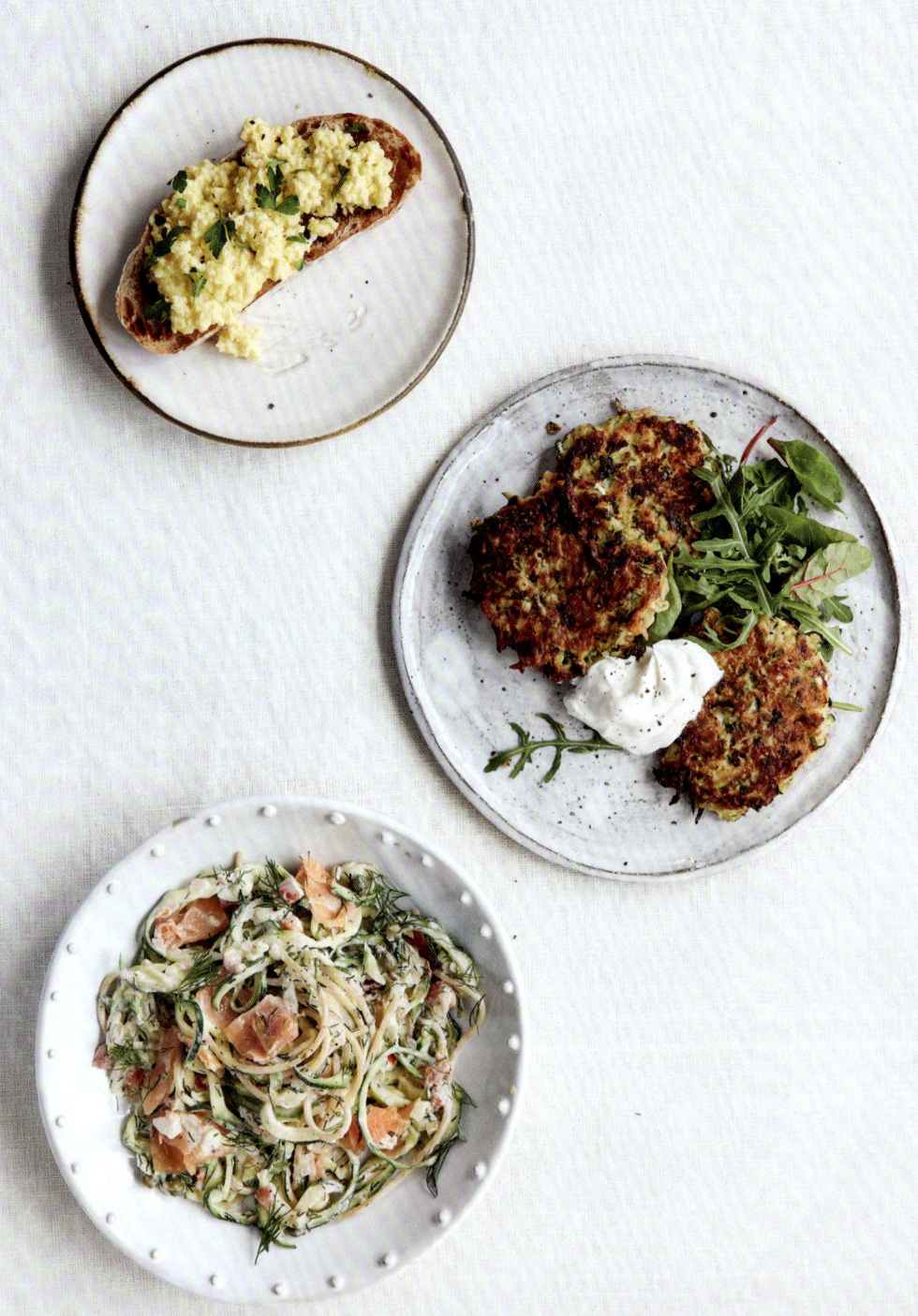

## Day 3
**Baked eggs with feta and spinach** (page 176)
**Crunchy chicken salad with blue cheese dressing** (page 189)
**Black pepper beef and veg stir fry** (page 219)

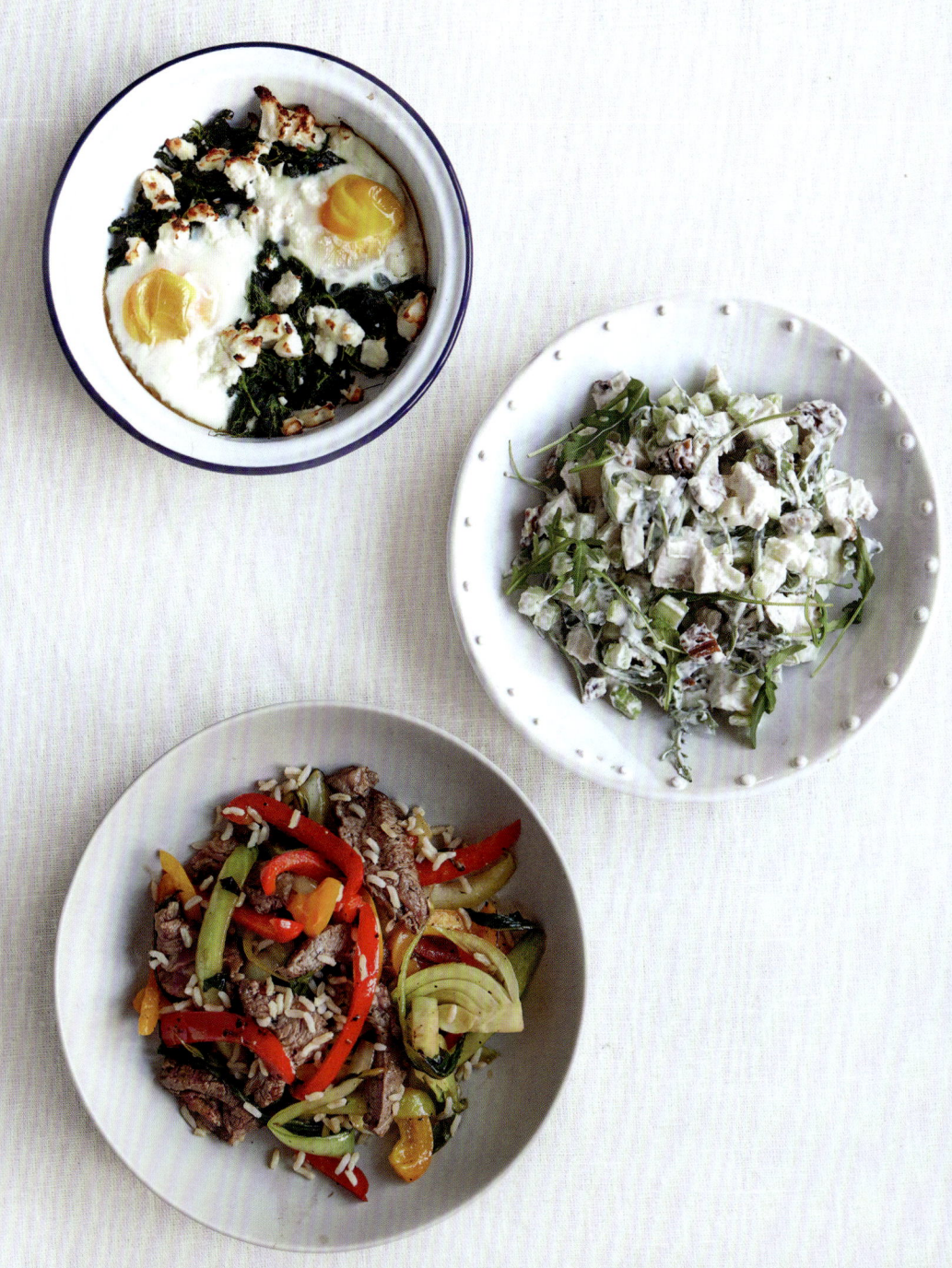

**Day 4**
Cherry tomato and haricot bean bake (page 178)
Greek spinach and feta pie (pages 193–4)
One pot chicken with chickpeas, garlic and thyme (page 203)

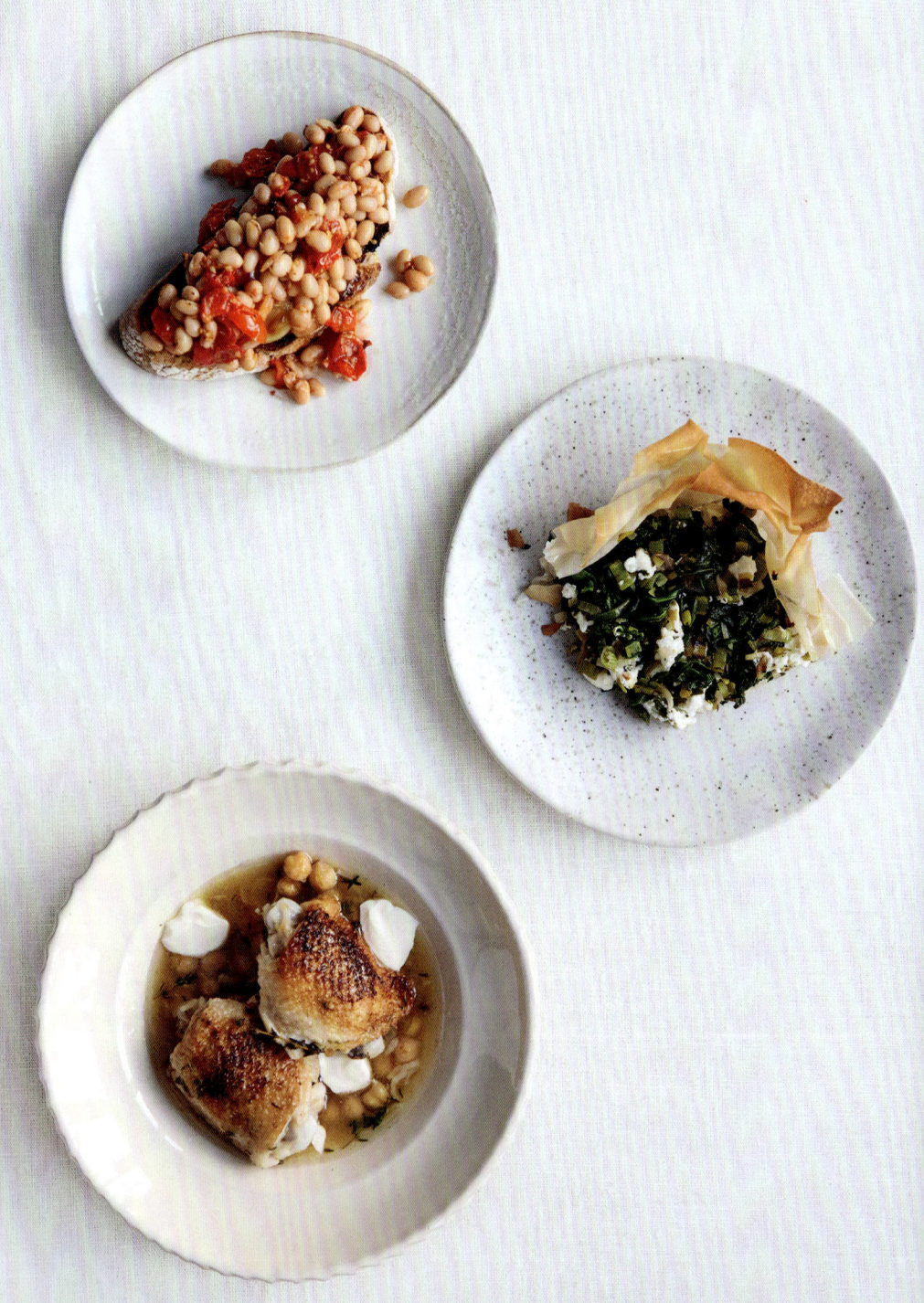

## Day 5
**Green shakshuka** (pages 171–2)
**Simple chowder** (pages 183–4)
**Black bean chilli with butternut squash and spinach** (pages 199–200)

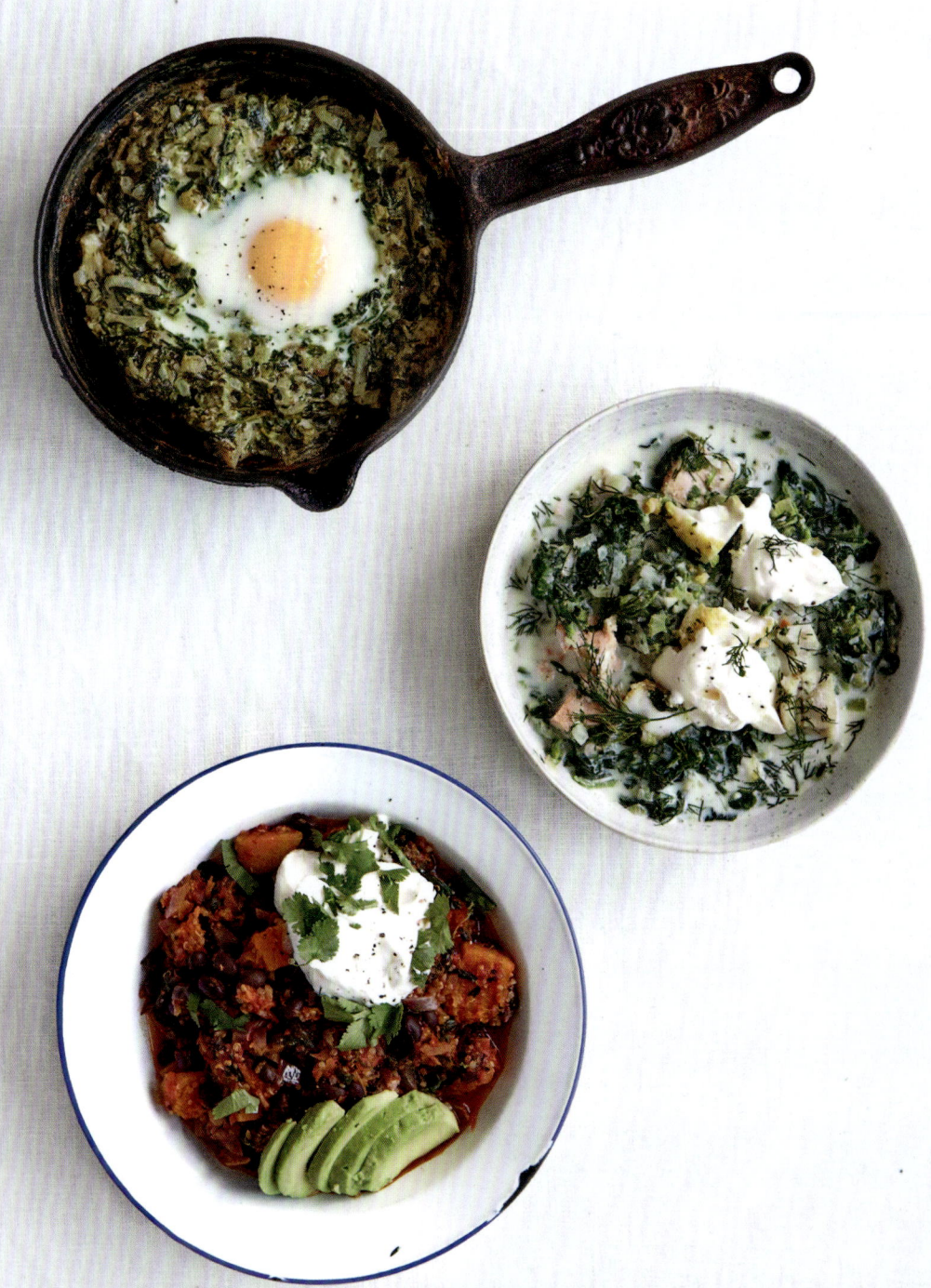

**Day 6**
Salmon and rocket egg muffins (page 173)
Mackerel and beetroot salad (page 186)
Trapanese courgetti pasta (pages 223–4)

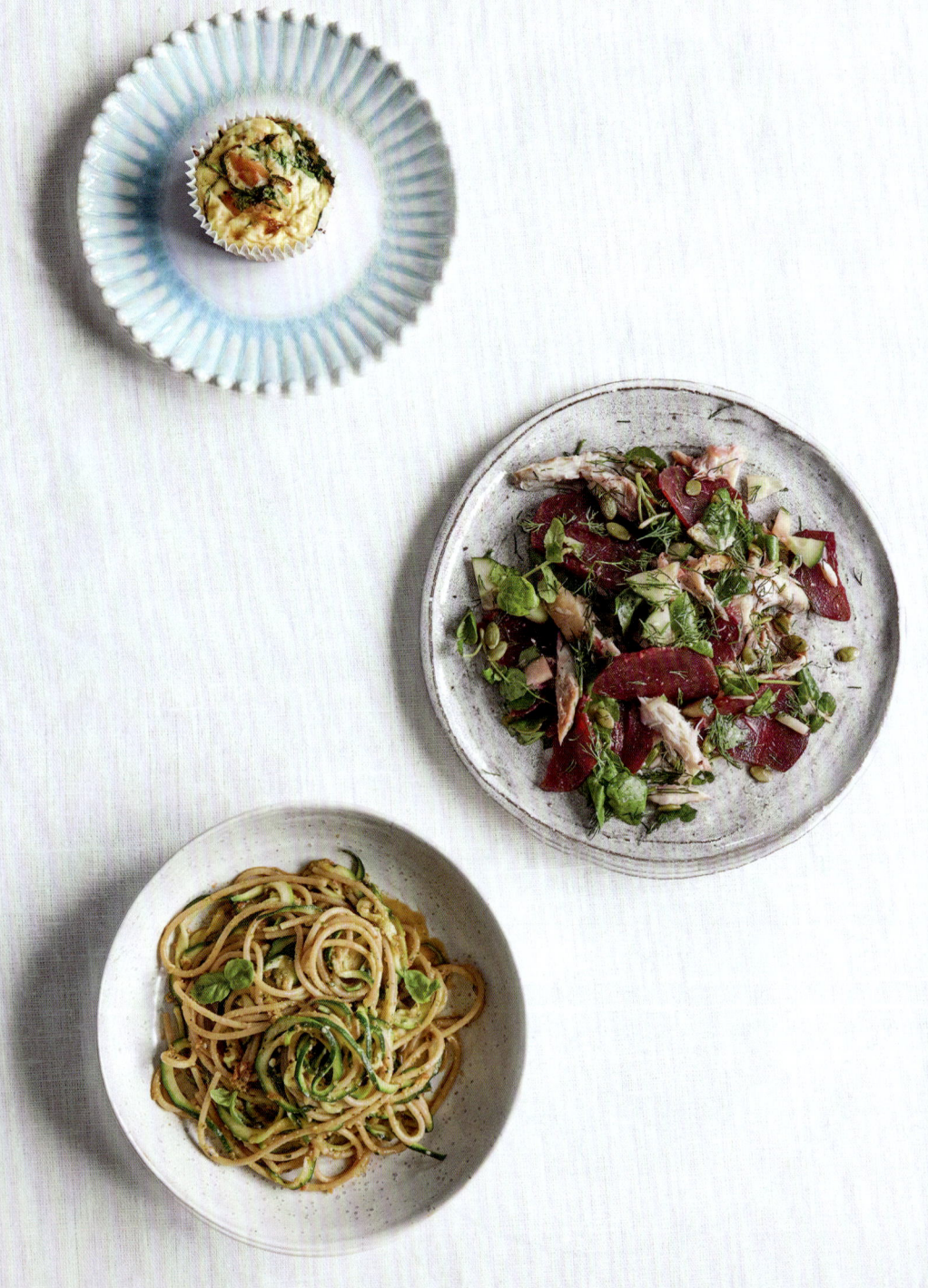

**Day 7**
Mushrooms on toast (page 179)
Smashed chilli avocado with fried egg and sauerkraut (page 185)
Gut-friendly shepherd's pie (pages 209–10)

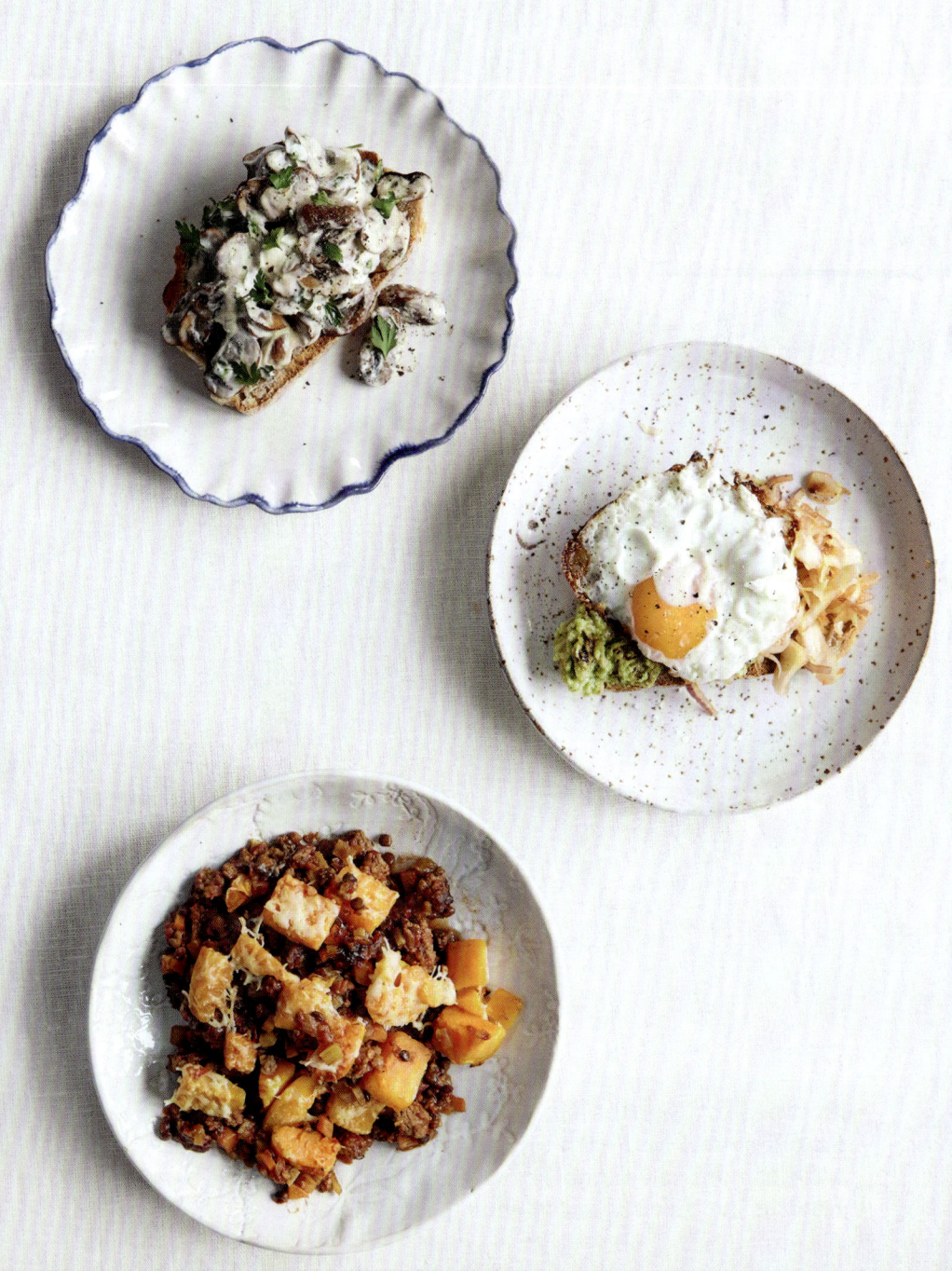

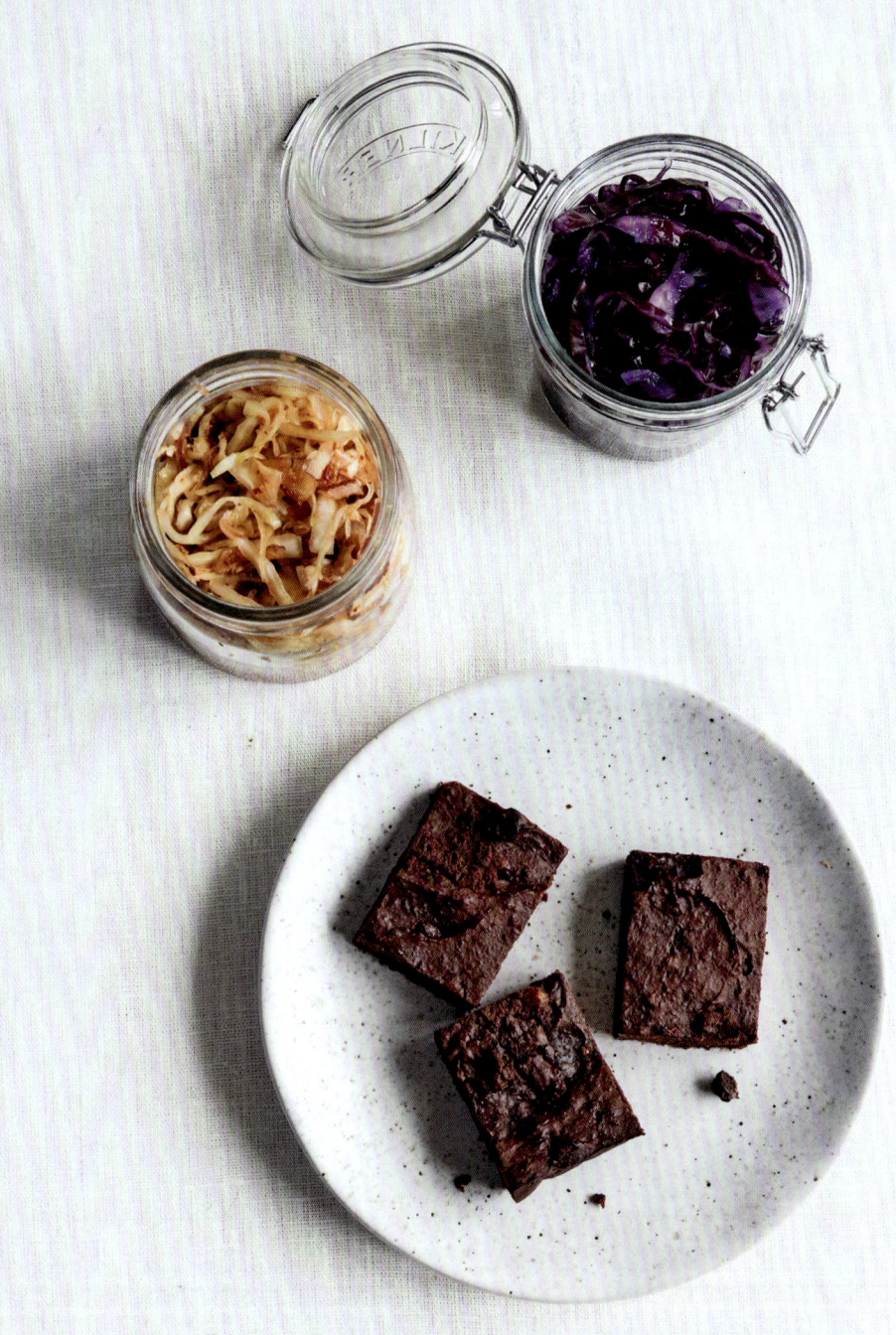

## Recipes for gut health

PART 4

# THE RECIPES

# Mango and lime chia pots

Light and zingy, with protein and fibre, this recipe serves two, but the pots will keep for a few days, making it a good one to prepare ahead.

Serves 2
Prep time: 5 mins

30g chia seeds
100g full-fat Greek yoghurt
120ml full-fat milk
50g mango
Zest of ½ lime
1 tbsp flaked almonds (optional)

1. Place all the ingredients except the almonds in a bowl. Blitz for about 30 seconds with a hand-held stick blender, being careful to retain some of the texture of the chia seeds.

2. Divide between two glasses and leave to set for about 30 minutes.

3. Top with the flaked almonds, if using, to serve.

**Nutrition per serving:** 174 calories / 9g protein / 6.5g fibre

# Nut butter and banana porridge

Porridge is a great source of fibre and acts as a prebiotic, too. To help you stay full for longer and get your morning protein, we have added milk and nut butter to power you through . . .

Serves 1
Prep time: 2 mins
Cook time: 5 mins

50g jumbo porridge oats
270ml full-fat milk or unsweetened nut milk
½ tsp ground cinnamon
1 tsp nut butter, such as almond butter
½ banana, peeled and roughly chopped

1. Place the oats in a small saucepan and pour in the milk. Add a pinch of salt and the cinnamon, and bring to the boil. Reduce the heat and simmer for 4–5 minutes, stirring often.

2. Remove from the heat and leave to cool for a couple of minutes.

3. Stir in the nut butter and chopped bananas, then tip into a bowl to serve.

**Nutrition per serving:** 448 calories / 16.5g protein / 5g fibre

# Green shakshuka

This shakshuka steps away from the traditional tomato base and uses delicious green veg instead. Perfect for a weekend brunch.

Serves 1

Prep time: 5 mins

Cook time: 15 mins

1 tbsp olive oil

½ onion, peeled and finely chopped

1 garlic clove, peeled and finely chopped

100g frozen spinach, defrosted and excess water squeezed out

2 tbsp full-fat cream cheese

¼ tsp grated nutmeg

1 medium free-range egg

1. Preheat the oven to 200°C/180°C Fan/Gas 6.

2. Place the olive oil in a small ovenproof frying pan over a medium heat. Add the onions and garlic and sauté for 2–3 minutes, until soft and translucent.

3. Add the spinach and heat through. Follow with the cream cheese, nutmeg and 2 tablespoons of water. Mix everything together well and season with salt and freshly ground black pepper. When the mixture is gently bubbling, make a well in the centre and crack in the egg.

4. Transfer the pan to the oven for 6–8 minutes, or until the egg whites are just set and the yolk is still runny. (Leave a little longer if you prefer your yolk firm.) Serve immediately.

**Nutrition per serving**: 310 calories / 13g protein / 4.5g fibre

## Salmon and rocket egg muffins

Bursting with protein and omega-3 in the salmon, this is brain food, too. Silicone muffin cases work best here, or a silicone muffin tray. All sorts of different veg and cheeses can be added to the basic milk mixture, making this a good recipe to use up leftovers in the fridge. Two muffins would make a substantial breakfast – the rest will keep in the fridge for a day or two. They also make a great daytime snack.

Makes 6

Prep time: 8 mins

Cook time: 15–18 mins

> 4 medium free-range eggs
> 50ml full-fat milk
> 100g smoked salmon
> 15g rocket, finely chopped
> Zest of ½ lemon

1. Preheat the oven to 200°C/180°C Fan/Gas 6. Place 6 silicone muffin cases or a silicone muffin tray on a baking tray for stability.

2. Whisk the eggs with the milk and season with salt and freshly ground black pepper. Stir in the smoked salmon, rocket and lemon zest.

3. Pour the mixture into the muffin cases or tray, then bake in the oven for 15–18 minutes or until set.

**Nutrition per serving:** 90 calories / 5.5g protein / 0g fibre

# Smoked salmon with avocado and tomatoes

An easy breakfast classic – rich in slow-burn, healthy fats that are needed to keep you full for longer and to support your important fat-soluble vitamins – A, D, E and K. You might like to add a piece of wholegrain or seeded sourdough for extra fibre.

Serves 1

Prep time: 5 mins

Cook time: 7 mins

> 1 medium free-range egg (optional)
> 1 small avocado, peeled, destoned and cut into 8 chunks
>   (100g prepared weight)
> Squeeze of fresh lemon juice
> 1 medium tomato, cut into 8 chunks (90g prepared weight)
> 1 tsp capers (optional)
> 1 tsp olive oil
> 2 slices smoked salmon (approx. 45g)

1. Place a small saucepan of water over a high heat and bring to the boil. Carefully lower in the egg and cook for 7 minutes. Remove the egg from the pan and run it under cold water. Peel, then cut the egg into quarters.

2. Toss the avocado with the lemon juice and place in a bowl with the tomato, capers (if using) and oil. Season with salt and freshly ground black pepper and toss together.

3. Serve the salad on a plate, topped with the smoked salmon and egg, if using.

**Nutrition per serving**: 325 calories / 14g protein / 5.5g fibre

# Baked eggs with feta and spinach

This is fast food for breakfast!

Serves 1
Prep time: 3 mins
Cook time: 8–10 mins

100g frozen spinach
2 medium free-range eggs
30g feta cheese, crumbled

1. Preheat the oven to 200°C/180°C Fan/Gas 6. You will need an 18cm round ovenproof dish.

2. Place the spinach in a microwaveable bowl and defrost in the microwave for 1–2 minutes. Leave to cool slightly, then squeeze out any excess water.

3. Place the spinach in the ovenproof dish, then the eggs and finally the feta cheese. Season with salt and bake in the oven for 8–10 minutes, or until the egg whites are set and the yolk is still runny. Sprinkle with freshly ground black pepper to serve.

**Nutrition per serving:** 260 calories / 23g protein / 3g fibre

# Omelette with ham, peas and Parmesan

So simple, this is ideal for using up leftover peas. Lots of lovely protein.

Serves 1
Prep time: 5 mins
Cook time: 2–3 mins

2 medium free-range eggs
½ tbsp olive oil
1 slice good-quality cooked ham, cut into 1cm dice
(30g prepared weight)
25g frozen peas, defrosted
2 tbsp finely grated Parmesan

1. Crack the eggs into a small bowl and whisk with a fork. Season with a pinch of salt and some freshly ground black pepper.

2. Place the olive oil in a non-stick frying pan over a medium heat. When hot, pour in the eggs. Leave for 30 seconds to start to set, then use a wooden spoon or spatula to pull the egg into the centre of the pan, allowing the runny mixture to flow out into the empty space – tilting the pan helps with this. Do this four or five times, working quite quickly.

3. Scatter the ham, peas and Parmesan all over the surface of the omelette, then fold one half over the other. Cook for a final minute, then slide on to a plate to serve.

**Nutrition per serving:** 356 calories / 31g protein / 1g fibre

# Cherry tomato and haricot bean bake

Delicious, garlicky white beans, full of fibre that your gut microbes will adore.

Serves 2
Prep time: 5 mins
Cook time: 25 mins

200g cherry tomatoes, halved
2 garlic cloves, peeled and left whole
2 tbsp olive oil
½ × 400g tin haricot beans, drained and rinsed (115g drained weight)
Pinch of dried chilli flakes (optional)
1 slice of seeded or wholemeal sourdough bread, toasted (optional)

1. Preheat the oven to 200°C/180°C Fan/Gas 6. You will need an ovenproof dish approximately 12.5 × 20cm in size.

2. Place the tomatoes and garlic in the base of the dish. Toss with the olive oil and bake in the oven for 20 minutes.

3. Add the haricot beans and return to the oven for a further 5 minutes.

4. Mix everything together and season with the chilli flakes, some salt and freshly ground black pepper. Serve with some sourdough toast, if using.

**Nutrition per serving**: 189 calories / 5g protein / 6g fibre

# Mushrooms on toast

Luxurious comfort food, and so easy and satisfying, too.

Serves 1

Prep time: 5 mins

Cook time: 7 mins

150g mushrooms, sliced

1 tbsp olive oil

1 tbsp full-fat crème fraîche

4 sprigs of parsley, leaves picked and roughly chopped

¼ tsp Dijon mustard (optional)

1 slice of seeded or wholemeal sourdough bread, toasted

1. Place the mushrooms and oil in a saucepan over a medium heat. Sauté the mushrooms for 5–6 minutes, or until they are soft and golden brown.

2. Remove the pan from the heat and stir in the crème fraîche, parsley and mustard, if using. Season with salt and freshly ground black pepper. Serve on top of the sourdough toast.

**Nutrition per serving**: 272 calories / 5.5g protein / 3g fibre

# Scrambled egg, Marmite and sourdough

There are benefits to sourdough, as it has been fermented, so it is more digestible and contains prebiotics, which are so important for gut health.

Serves 1
Prep time: 2 mins
Cook time: 3 mins

1 tsp olive oil
1 medium free-range egg
1 tsp Marmite
1 slice of seeded or wholemeal sourdough bread, toasted
2 sprigs of parsley, leaves picked and roughly chopped (optional)

1.  Place the olive oil in a small frying pan over a medium heat. When hot, crack in the egg and fry for about 2 minutes, or until the egg is crispy around the edges, the whites are set and the yolk is still runny (cook for longer if you prefer it firmer). Remove from the heat.

2.  Spread the Marmite onto the toast, top with the fried egg and garnish with parsley, if using. Season with freshly ground black pepper and serve.

**Nutrition per serving:** 215 calories / 13g protein / 3g fibre

## Quick spinach and pea soup

Simple comfort food, packed with anti-inflammatory polyphenols.

Serves 2
Prep time: 5 mins
Cook time: 6–8 mins

1½ tbsp olive oil
1 small leek, trimmed and roughly sliced
500ml vegetable or chicken stock
150g frozen peas
150g frozen spinach

1. Heat the olive oil in a saucepan over a medium heat and sauté the leeks for 3 minutes, or until softened.

2. Add the vegetable stock, peas and spinach, and bring to the boil. Cover with a lid, reduce the heat and simmer for 3 minutes.

3. Remove the soup from the heat and use a hand-held blender to blitz until smooth. Season with salt and freshly ground black pepper to taste.

## Note

For extra flavour, add 1–2 teaspoons of pesto, and for extra protein stir in 1 tablespoon of Greek yoghurt, or crumble in some feta.

**Nutrition per serving**: 204 calories / 9g protein / 9g fibre

# Simple chowder

Get your omega-3 fix with this fabulous, protein-rich, thick fish soup.

Serves 4

Prep time: 10 mins

Cook time: 15 mins

  1 medium onion, peeled and finely chopped

  2 sticks of celery, finely chopped (80g prepared weight)

  1 tbsp olive oil

  2 garlic cloves, peeled and finely chopped

  400ml veg or chicken stock

  150g frozen spinach

  400ml full-fat milk

  340g fish pie mix (e.g. salmon, cod and smoked haddock)

  7g fresh dill, finely chopped

  2 tbsp full-fat crème fraîche (optional)

1. Place the onion, celery and olive oil in a saucepan over a medium heat. Sauté for 3–4 minutes, until softened. Add the garlic and sauté for another minute.

2. Pour in the stock and add the spinach. Bring to the boil, then reduce the heat and simmer for 3 minutes.

3. Pour in the milk, add the fish pie mix and poach over a low heat for 5 minutes. It is important not to boil the chowder at this point, or it will split.

4. Finally, stir in the dill and crème fraîche, if using, and season with salt and freshly ground black pepper to serve.

**Nutrition per serving**: 232 calories / 25g protein / 3g fibre

# Smashed chilli avocado
# with fried egg and sauerkraut

The sauerkraut adds an extra sweet and tangy flavour, and boosts your gut microbiome. This, in turn, helps support immunity, reduces inflammation and even improves mood. Why not try making your own (page 247)?

Serves 1

Prep time: 2 mins

Cook time: 2–3 mins

½ avocado, flesh scooped out (60g prepared weight)

¼ tsp dried chilli flakes

1 tsp olive oil

1 medium free-range egg

1 slice of seeded or wholemeal sourdough bread, toasted

1 tbsp sauerkraut (shop bought or see page 247)

1. Mash the avocado with the chilli flakes and a pinch of salt and freshly ground black pepper, then set aside.

2. Heat the olive oil in a small frying pan over a medium heat. Crack the egg into the pan and fry for about 2–3 minutes, or until the egg is crispy around the edges, the whites are set and the yolk is still runny (cook for longer if you prefer it firmer). Remove from the heat.

3. Spread the smashed avocado on the sourdough, top with the fried egg and sauerkraut, season to taste and serve.

**Nutrition per serving:** 324 calories / 13g protein / 6g fibre

# Mackerel and beetroot salad

Mackerel is a good source of much-needed omega-3. This colourful, easy-to-assemble salad has a sweet and mustardy dressing and plenty of crunch. Any nuts or seeds will work in this recipe, and you can also use whatever mustard you like.

Serves 2
Prep time: 7 mins

70g watercress or rocket
10g fresh dill, roughly chopped
1 cooked beetroot (approx. 120g), thinly sliced
2 cooked mackerel fillets (approx. 200g), skin removed and flaked
¼ cucumber, roughly chopped
1 tbsp pumpkin seeds (10g)
¾ tbsp Dijon mustard
1 tbsp apple cider vinegar
1½ tbsp olive oil

1. Arrange the watercress or rocket, dill, beetroot, mackerel, cucumber and pumpkin seeds in a bowl.

2. Place the mustard, vinegar and oil in a small bowl with a pinch of salt and freshly ground black pepper. Whisk until emulsified.

3. Pour all over the salad, toss to coat, then divide between two plates to serve.

**Nutrition per serving:** 442 calories / 25g protein / 3g fibre

# Sardine, avocado and rocket salad with chilli dressing and sourdough croutons

More super-healthy oily fish, brought to life with chilli flakes and a dash of apple cider vinegar.

Serves 2

Prep time: 10 mins

Cook time: 5 mins

1 slice of sourdough bread (50g), cut into 1cm cubes

2 tbsp olive oil

1 tsp dried chilli flakes

1 tbsp apple cider vinegar

2 heads of baby gem lettuce, shredded

2 medium tomatoes, each cut into 8 (approx. 180g)

1 small avocado, peeled, destoned and cut into 8

2 × 100g tins sardines in olive oil, drained

1. Preheat the oven to 200°C/180°C Fan/Gas 6.

2. Toss the sourdough cubes with 1 tablespoon of the olive oil and a pinch of salt and freshly ground black pepper. Spread out on a baking tray and place in the oven for 5 minutes, or until golden and crisp.

3. Mix the remaining olive oil with the chilli flakes and apple cider vinegar in a small bowl. Season with a pinch of salt and pepper and mix well together.

4. Arrange the baby gem, tomatoes and avocado on a plate and pour the dressing all over. Toss to coat thoroughly. Place the sardines and croutons on top and serve.

**Nutrition per serving:** 472 calories / 25g protein / 5g fibre

# Crunchy chicken salad with blue cheese dressing

Ideal for using up leftover chicken for a quick, protein-rich lunch, or to take to work in a lunchbox.

Serves 2

Prep time: 10 mins

Cook time: 5 mins

½ green apple, finely diced (40g prepared weight)

1 tbsp fresh lemon juice, plus 1 tsp

2 sticks of celery, finely chopped (80g prepared weight)

25g rocket, finely chopped

20g pecan nuts, roughly chopped

150g cooked chicken, roughly chopped

3 tbsp full-fat Greek yoghurt

40g gorgonzola cheese

1.  Place the apple in a bowl with 1 teaspoon of the lemon juice and toss to coat. Add the celery, rocket, pecans and the chicken.

2.  In a separate bowl, mash the yoghurt with the remaining lemon juice and the gorgonzola until smooth. Season with a pinch of salt and freshly ground black pepper.

3.  Pour over the salad and toss to thoroughly coat, then serve.

**Nutrition per serving**: 308 calories / 30g protein / 2g fibre

# Curried chicken open sandwich with rocket

Perfect for a quick but filling lunch with lots of flavour.

Serves 1
Prep time: 7 mins

- 100g cooked chicken, finely chopped
- 2 tbsp full-fat Greek yoghurt
- ¾ tsp curry powder
- 1 slice of sourdough bread, toasted
- ½ tsp olive oil
- Small handful of rocket (approx.10g)

1. Mix the chicken with the yoghurt, curry powder and a pinch of salt and freshly ground black pepper.

2. Drizzle the sourdough toast with the olive oil. Top with the rocket and curried chicken to serve.

**Note**

To make this more portable and to keep bread to a minimum, serve the chicken in a seeded wrap. It'll make a great lunchbox filler!

**Nutrition per serving:** 324 calories / 36.5g protein / 2g fibre

# Courgette and carrot fritters with coriander

These tangy and flavourful fritters also make a filling and portable meal, or they can accompany another dish.

Serves 2

Prep time: 10 mins

Cook time: 5 mins

1 small courgette (approx. 120g), coarsely grated

1 small carrot (approx. 70g), coarsely grated

80g feta cheese, crumbled

20g fresh coriander, roughly chopped

2 tbsp flour, such as spelt, wholegrain or buckwheat flour

2 medium free-range eggs

1 tbsp olive oil

1.  Mix the grated courgette and carrot in a bowl with the feta, coriander, flour, eggs and a generous pinch of salt and freshly ground pepper until thoroughly combined.

2.  Place ½ tablespoon of the olive oil in a non-stick frying pan over a medium heat. When hot, add 3 spoonfuls of the courgette and carrot mixture into the pan and fry for 2 minutes. Carefully flip over each fritter and fry for 1½ minutes on the other side. Remove from the pan and keep warm. Repeat with the remaining olive oil and fritter mixture. You should have 6 fritters in total.

3. Serve them on their own, or with a spoonful of Greek yoghurt and a little green salad on the side.

**Nutrition per serving:** 309 calories / 17g protein / 3.5g fibre

# Greek spinach and feta pie

This simple-to-make filo pie is scrumptious straight out of the oven, or eaten cold for an 'on the go' lunch. It can also hold its own simply with a dressed green salad. Made using thin filo pastry, it remains relatively low in starchy carbohydrates, and with all that spinach it is positively overflowing with healthy nutrients.

Serves 4
Prep time: 10 mins
Cook time: 30 mins

   3 tbsp olive oil
   1 leek, trimmed, quartered lengthwise and finely sliced
   200g frozen spinach
   100g feta cheese, crumbled
   2 sheets of filo pastry

1. Preheat the oven to 220°C/200°C Fan/Gas 7. Line a baking tray with parchment paper.

2. Place 1 tablespoon of the olive oil in a frying pan over a medium heat. When hot, add the leeks and sauté for 3–4 minutes, or until soft. Add a tablespoon of water halfway through the cooking time to help the process along.

3. Meanwhile, place the spinach in a microwaveable bowl and cook in the microwave for 2–3 minutes. When defrosted, transfer to a sieve and press out as much excess water as possible.

4. Add the spinach to the pan with the leeks and heat through for 2 minutes. Stir in the feta, season with salt and freshly ground black pepper, then set aside.

5. Lay one sheet of filo pastry on the prepared baking tray. Brush some oil over the surface of the pastry, then place the second sheet of filo on top. Brush this with olive oil also. Spoon the spinach mixture into the centre of the pastry and spread out, making sure to leave a border 5cm from each edge. Pull the edges up and scrunch together, to create a pie with a frilled top. Brush the edges with the remaining oil and bake in the oven for 20 minutes, until golden and crisp. Serve on its own or with a green salad.

**Nutrition per serving:** 194 calories / 7g protein / 3g fibre

# Grilled cheese on seeded bread with sauerkraut

A fabulously easy, gut-friendly variation of cheese on toast.

Serves 1
Prep time: 5 mins
Cook time: 2–3 mins

 35g frozen spinach
 1 tsp Dijon mustard
 50g Cheddar, coarsely grated
 1 slice of seeded bread, lightly toasted
 1 tbsp sauerkraut (shop bought or see page 247)

1. Preheat the grill to high.

2. Place the spinach in the microwaveable bowl and cook for about 1 minute, until defrosted. Leave to cool a little, then squeeze out all the excess water. Place in a clean bowl and mix with the mustard and grated cheese, and season with salt and freshly ground black pepper.

3. Spread on the toast and place under the grill for 3–4 minutes, or until bubbling and golden.

4. Top with sauerkraut to serve.

**Nutrition per serving:** 360 calories / 19g protein / 4.5g fibre

# Seeded wrap with smoked salmon, capers and cream cheese

A satisfying and classic combo in a wrap.

Serves 1

Prep time: 8 mins

- 1 medium seeded tortilla wrap
- 2 tbsp full-fat cream cheese (30g)
- 4 baby gem leaves, roughly sliced (30g)
- ½ medium tomato, sliced (40g)
- 2 small slices of smoked salmon (45g)
- 1 tsp capers

1. Place the tortilla on top of a toaster and turn on the heat. Flip the tortilla a few times, as it begins to heat through and turns golden. After a minute or so, remove the wrap and put on a plate.

2. Spread the cream cheese over the wrap, then top with the lettuce, tomato, smoked salmon and capers. Season with salt and freshly ground black pepper. Fold in half to serve.

**Nutrition per serving**: 384 calories / 19g protein / 4g fibre

# Rye bread with hummus, pesto and a fried egg

A winning combination of Nordic and Mediterranean flavours – both cuisines known for healthy food.

Serves 1

Prep time: 2 mins

Cook time: 2–3 mins

  1 tsp olive oil

  1 medium free-range egg

  1 tbsp good-quality basil pesto

  1 slice of rye bread, toasted

  1 tbsp hummus

1. Place the olive oil in a small frying pan over a medium heat. When hot, crack in the egg and fry for 2–3 minutes, or until the egg is crispy around the edges, the whites are set and the yolk is still runny (cook for longer if you prefer it firmer). Remove from the heat.

2. Spread the pesto on to the toast, then the hummus. Top with the egg, and season with salt and freshly ground black pepper to serve.

**Nutrition per serving:** 326 calories / 12.5g protein / 3g fibre

# Black bean chilli with butternut squash and spinach

This is a feisty favourite in our family, full of gut-friendly beans and fibre. All but a few ingredients are from the store cupboard. It can easily be scaled up for parties.

Serves 2
Prep time: 10 mins
Cook time: 30 mins

1 tbsp olive oil
1 medium red onion, peeled and finely chopped
3 garlic cloves, peeled and roughly chopped
1 tsp smoked sweet paprika
1 tsp ground cumin
½ tsp cayenne pepper
1 × 400g tin chopped tomatoes
1 × 400g tin black beans, drained and rinsed
200g butternut squash (fresh or frozen),
 peeled and cut into chunks
100g frozen spinach

1. Place the olive oil in a saucepan over a medium heat. When hot, add the onions and sauté for 3 minutes, stirring from time to time. Add the garlic and cook for 1 minute.

2. Stir in the spices, chopped tomatoes, black beans, squash and 400ml water, and bring to the boil. Cover with a lid, reduce the heat and simmer for 15 minutes.

3. Stir in the frozen spinach and cook for a final 5 minutes.

4. You could serve this with full-fat Greek or coconut yoghurt, sliced avocado, fresh coriander and 2–3 tablespoons of quinoa, too.

**Nutrition per serving**: 292 calories / 14.5g protein / 19.5g fibre

# Roasted salmon and courgettes with anchovy chilli butter

This is so simple and full of flavour, thanks to the anchovies, which also deliver some more omega -3.

Serves 2

Prep time: 5 mins

Cook time: 17 mins

> 2 medium courgettes (approx. 500g), sliced into 1cm rounds
>
> 1 tbsp olive oil
>
> 2 salmon fillets (approx. 240g combined weight)
>
> 35g butter, softened
>
> 3 anchovy fillets, finely chopped
>
> 1 garlic clove, peeled and finely grated

1. Preheat the oven to 200°C/180°C Fan/Gas 6. Line a baking tray with parchment paper.

2. Lay the courgettes on the baking tray, drizzle with the olive oil and season with salt and freshly ground black pepper. Roast in the oven for 5 minutes.

3. Carefully remove the tray from the oven and place the salmon fillets in between the courgettes. Return to the oven for 10 minutes.

4. Meanwhile, place the butter, anchovies and garlic in a small bowl and mash them together.

5. Remove the baking tray once more, spoon the anchovy butter over the salmon and return to the oven for a final 2 minutes.

6. Serve with 2–3 heaped tablespoons of quinoa or brown rice.

**Nutrition per serving:** 501 calories / 30.5g protein / 3.5g fibre

# One pot chicken with chickpeas, garlic and thyme

Easy comfort food that you and your gut microbiome will love, thanks to the chickpeas and roasted garlic, and not to mention all that much-needed protein!

Serves 4

Prep time: 10 mins

Cook time: 45 mins

2 tbsp olive oil

8 skin on, bone in chicken thighs (approx. 1.2kg)

3 garlic cloves, peeled and roughly chopped, plus 1 whole head of garlic, top sliced off

2 × 400g tins chickpeas, drained

6 sprigs of thyme, leaves picked and chopped, plus 2 extra sprigs (or 2 tsp dried thyme)

400ml chicken stock

2 tbsp crème fraîche

1. Preheat the oven to 180°C/160°C Fan/Gas 4.

2. Place the olive oil in a heavy-based ovenproof lidded saucepan over a medium heat. When hot, lay the chicken in the pan, skin side down. Sear for 3–4 minutes, or until the skin is golden and crisp. Remove from the pan and set aside.

3. Reduce the heat, add the chopped garlic and fry for 30 seconds. Stir in the chickpeas and chopped thyme and season with salt and freshly ground black pepper. Heat through.

4. Pour in the stock and return the chicken to the pan, skin side up. Place the head of garlic and remaining sprigs of thyme among the chicken, then bring the pan to the boil. Cover with a lid and transfer to the oven for 40 minutes, until the chicken is cooked through.

5. Serve with the crème fraîche and 2–3 tablespoons of bulgur wheat or brown rice.

**Nutrition per serving**: 510 calories / 54g protein / 8g fibre

# Aubergine, tomato and mozzarella bake

Mediterranean-style comfort food.

Serves 2

Prep time: 15 mins

Cook time: 40 mins

1 × 400g tin haricot beans, drained

2 tbsp olive oil

1½ tsp dried oregano

1 medium aubergine (approx. 300g), sliced into 1cm half moons

3 tomatoes (approx. 200g), each sliced into 5

2 × 125g balls of mozzarella, drained and each sliced into 8

1. Preheat the oven to 200°C/180°C Fan/Gas 6. You will need a 20cm square baking dish.

2. Tip the haricot beans into the base of the baking dish with 1 tablespoon of the olive oil and 1 teaspoon of the oregano. Season with salt and freshly ground black pepper and mix well.

3. Arrange the slices of aubergine, tomato and mozzarella on top. Start with a slice of aubergine, followed by a slice of tomato, then mozzarella, and continue until the surface of the beans is more or less covered.

4. Drizzle the remaining olive oil on top and sprinkle with the remaining oregano, as well as a final pinch of salt and pepper.

5.  Bake in the oven for 35–40 minutes, or until the aubergines are golden and the sauce is bubbling.

**Nutrition per serving**: 600 calories / 33.5g protein / 15g fibre

# Very mild prawn and cashew curry

The main work for this dish is in the preparation – the rest of it comes together in minutes. It is bound to become a favourite. White fish, such as cod, or even salmon, could be used instead of prawns.

Serves 2
Prep time: 15 mins
Cook time: 8 mins

  1 tbsp olive oil
  1 medium onion, peeled and finely chopped
  2 garlic cloves, peeled and finely chopped
  1 red chilli, deseeded and finely chopped
  2.5cm piece of fresh root ginger, peeled and coarsely grated
  1 tsp ground turmeric (optional)
  1 tbsp mild curry powder
  1 × 400g tin coconut milk
  50g cashew nuts
  250g frozen king prawns, defrosted
  Small handful of fresh coriander (approx. 10g),
    roughly chopped (optional)

1. Place the olive oil in a saucepan over a medium heat. When hot, add the onion and sauté for 2–3 minutes. Add the garlic, chilli and ginger, and cook for 1 minute, stirring all the time.

2. Add the turmeric, if using, and curry powder, and heat through for about 20 seconds. Pour in the coconut milk, and add the cashews and prawns. Stir well and bring to the boil. Reduce the heat and simmer for 1 minute.

3. Remove from the heat, stir in the coriander, if using, and serve with 2–3 tablespoons of brown rice.

**Nutrition per serving**: 669 calories / 25g protein / 6g fibre

# Gut-friendly shepherd's pie

For good gut health we are encouraged to eat 30 or more plants a week. This delivers almost 10 in one sitting! The more variety of plants we eat, the more of their different nutrients you benefit from.

Serves 4

Prep time: 15 mins

Cook time: 45 mins

2 tbsp olive oil

1 medium onion, peeled and finely chopped

2 carrots, peeled and diced (150g prepared weight)

2 sticks of celery, trimmed and diced (100g prepared weight)

3 garlic cloves, peeled and roughly chopped

3 sprigs of thyme, leaves picked, or 1 tsp dried thyme (optional)

250g minced beef

1 beef stock cube

1 × 400g tin chopped tomatoes

1 tsp paprika (optional)

1½ tbsp Worcestershire sauce

150g cooked Puy lentils

350g butternut squash (fresh or frozen), peeled and
    cut into chunks

50g Cheddar, grated

1. Preheat the oven to 220°C/200°C Fan/Gas 7.

2. Place the olive oil in a large lidded frying pan over a medium heat. When hot, add the onion and sauté for 2–3 minutes until soft. Add the carrot and celery and cook for 5 minutes with the lid on, stirring from time to time. Add the garlic and thyme, if using, and cook for 30 seconds.

3. Stir in the minced beef and use a wooden spoon to break it up into small pieces. Cook for about 3 minutes, until browned. Crumble in the stock cube and stir in the chopped tomatoes, 400ml water, the paprika, if using, and the Worcestershire sauce. Cover with a lid and simmer over a medium heat for 15 minutes.

4. Remove the lid and stir in the cooked Puy lentils. Remove from the heat, season with salt and freshly ground black pepper and transfer to the baking dish.

5. Top with the frozen butternut squash, and sprinkle over the Cheddar. Bake in the oven for 30 minutes, until the butternut squash is tender and the cheese is golden.

**Nutrition per serving:** 400 calories / 22.5g protein / 8g fibre

# Braised Puy lentils with grilled chicken

This is a brilliant, high fibre and protein dish. Puy lentils are slightly special as they tend to hold their shape and remain *al dente* when cooked. They are great to pad out a stew or Bolognese with extra fibre, while managing to go unnoticed for those who aren't lentil lovers.

Serves 2

Prep time: 25 mins

Cook time: 35–40 mins

2 tbsp olive oil

1 medium onion, peeled and finely chopped

1 medium carrot, peeled and diced (100g prepared weight)

1 stick of celery, trimmed and diced (50g prepared weight)

1 tsp dried thyme

150g dried Puy lentils

800ml chicken stock

2 skinless chicken breasts

1. Place 1 tablespoon of the olive oil in a saucepan over a medium heat. When hot, add the onion, carrot, celery and thyme, and sauté for 5 minutes. Add the Puy lentils and chicken stock, cover with a lid and simmer for 25–30 minutes. Season with salt and freshly ground black pepper.

2. Place the chicken breasts between two large pieces of parchment paper and bash with a rolling pin to flatten them. You want them to be roughly 1cm thick.

3. Heat the remaining oil in a large frying or griddle pan over a high heat, and cook the chicken for 3–4 minutes on each side. Remove from the heat and set aside to rest for a few minutes.

4. Serve each breast on a generous helping of Puy lentils.

**Nutrition per serving:** 603 calories / 65g protein / 13g fibre

# Baked cod with leeks, peas and white beans

A simple, creamy fish traybake with peas.

Serves 2

Prep time: 5 mins

Cook time: 15 mins

1 tbsp olive oil

1 medium leek, trimmed, halved lengthways and finely sliced (120g prepared weight)

1 × 400g tin white beans, such as haricot or cannellini, drained and rinsed

300ml vegetable stock

2 skinless cod fillets (280g combined weight)

100g frozen peas

2 tbsp full-fat crème fraîche

½ lemon, cut into wedges, to serve

1. Preheat the oven to 200°C/180°C Fan/Gas 6.

2. Place the olive oil in a shallow flameproof casserole over a medium heat. When hot, add the leek and sauté for 3–4 minutes, until soft.

3. Add the beans and stock and bring to the boil. Place the cod fillets on top and transfer to the oven for 12 minutes.

4. Carefully remove the dish from the oven, stir in the peas and season with salt and freshly ground black pepper. Return to the oven for 2 minutes.

5. Finally, remove the dish from the oven, stir in the crème fraîche, and serve with the lemon wedges for squeezing.

**Nutrition per serving**: 419 calories / 38g protein / 15g fibre

# One pot chicken with fennel and peppers

A Mediterranean whole chicken tray bake, with lots of colourful veg and plenty of protein.

Serves 4
Prep time: 10 mins
Cook time: 1 hr 10 mins

2 tbsp olive oil

1 whole chicken (approx. 1.4kg)

1 fennel bulb, sliced into 8 wedges lengthways, reserving the fronds (250g prepared weight)

3 medium peppers, any colour, deseeded and each sliced into 6 wedges (350g prepared weight)

300g cherry tomatoes

200ml chicken stock

50g pitted kalamata olives, roughly chopped

1. Preheat the oven to 200°C/180°C Fan/Gas 6.

2. Place 1 tablespoon of the olive oil in a large lidded flameproof casserole over a medium heat. Add the chicken, breast side down, and brown for 3–4 minutes.

3. Carefully turn the chicken over and add the fennel wedges, peppers and tomatoes around the chicken. Pour in the stock, season with salt and freshly ground black pepper, cover with a lid and transfer to the oven for 50 minutes.

4. Add the olives to the casserole, then return it to the oven to cook for a further 15–20 minutes, or until the juices of the chicken run clear. Leave the chicken to rest for about 5 minutes.

5. Garnish with the fennel fronds to serve.

**Nutrition per serving**: 384 calories / 51g protein / 5g fibre

# Pan-seared pork with tomatoes, balsamic and basil

The sweet tanginess of the balsamic vinegar cuts through the pork beautifully, and the recipe is so very quick and easy to make, too.

Serves 2

Prep time: 7 mins

Cook time: 16 mins

2 tbsp olive oil

2 pork chops (450g combined weight)

400g cherry tomatoes, halved

2 tbsp balsamic vinegar

3–4 sprigs of basil, leaves finely sliced

1. Preheat the oven to 200°C/180°C Fan/Gas 6.

2. Rub 1 tablespoon of the olive oil over the pork chops and season with a generous pinch of salt and freshly ground black pepper.

3. Place an ovenproof frying pan over a high heat. When really hot, add the pork chops and sear for 1½ minutes on each side. Turn them onto their fatty edges and move to one side of the pan.

4. Add the remaining oil and the tomatoes to the pan and fry for about 1 minute. Pour in the balsamic vinegar and place the pork chops flat on top of the tomatoes. Transfer to the oven for 12 minutes.

5. Remove the chops from the pan and stir the basil through the tomatoes. Check the seasoning. Serve with some baby new potatoes and steamed broccoli or greens.

**Nutrition per serving**: 577 calories / 73g protein / 2.5g fibre

# Black pepper beef and veg stir fry

This is one of my favourites – an aromatic stir fry with a very mild heat from the pepper, but not too spicy. Substitute tofu for beef to make this vegetarian.

Serves 2

Prep time: 10 mins

Cook time: 3–4 mins

> 1 × 250g rump steak, very thinly sliced
>
> 2 tsp freshly ground black pepper
>
> 1 tbsp soy sauce
>
> 1 tbsp oyster sauce
>
> 1 tbsp rice vinegar
>
> ½ tsp cornflour
>
> 1½ tbsp olive oil
>
> 2 medium peppers, any colour, deseeded and finely sliced
>     (275g prepared weight)
>
> 2 heads of pak choi, finely sliced (250g prepared weight)

1. Toss the sliced steak with 1 teaspoon of the black pepper and the salt. Place the remaining black pepper, soy sauce, oyster sauce, rice vinegar and cornflour in a small bowl and add 50ml water. Mix until the cornflour is dissolved.

2. Place the olive oil in a large frying pan or wok over a high heat. When smoking hot, add the steak and stir fry for about 45 seconds. Remove from the pan and set aside.

3. Add the peppers and pak choi to the pan and stir fry for 1½ minutes. Pour in the sauce and return the steak to the pan. Mix together and stir fry for about 30 seconds to allow the sauce to thicken.

4. Serve with 2–3 tablespoons of cooked brown rice or a small portion of egg noodles.

**Nutrition per serving**: 332 calories / 31g protein / 5.5g fibre

# Smoked salmon, dill and caper pasta

If you are cutting down the carbs and reducing your pasta, switch in some juicy, spiralised courgette for a win–win!

Serves 2

Prep time: 7 mins

Cook time: 8–10 mins

40g wholegrain spaghetti

2 courgettes, spiralised, or 300g shop-bought courgetti

1 tbsp olive oil

1 small onion, peeled and very finely chopped

1 medium tomato, finely chopped

1 tbsp capers

3 tbsp crème fraîche

100g smoked salmon, roughly chopped

10g fresh dill, finely chopped

1. Bring a pan of salted water to the boil and cook the pasta for 8 minutes, or until al dente. Remove from the heat and add the courgetti to the pan for 45 seconds to soften. Drain, reserving 4 tablespoons of the cooking water, and set the pasta and courgetti aside, keeping warm.

2. Place the olive oil in a frying pan over a medium heat. When hot, add the onion and sauté for 2 minutes, until softened. Add the tomato and capers, and cook for 2 minutes.

3. Turn off the heat and stir in the crème fraîche and the reserved cooking water to create a sauce. Add the smoked salmon and dill and season with salt and freshly ground black pepper. Mix well.

4. Add the pasta and courgetti to the pan and toss together well to coat. Serve immediately.

**Nutrition per serving:** 359 calories / 19g protein / 6g fibre

# Trapanese courgetti pasta

Trapanese pesto is a Sicilian pesto made with almonds, basil, garlic, tomatoes and Parmesan or pecorino cheese. It is full of flavour and texture.

Serves 2
Prep time: 10 mins
Cook time: 10 mins

20g blanched almonds

1 garlic clove, peeled

Bunch of basil (approx. 15g), leaves picked

20g Parmesan, roughly chopped

1 medium tomato, roughly chopped (90g prepared weight)

3 tbsp olive oil

40g wholegrain spaghetti

2 courgettes, spiralised, or 300g shop-bought courgetti

1. Place the almonds in a dry frying pan over a medium heat and toast for about 2 minutes, until golden brown. Transfer to a food processor, along with the garlic, basil leaves and Parmesan. Blitz until the nuts are roughly chopped. Add the tomato and olive oil and pulse a couple of times, until the tomatoes have just broken down but are still a bit chunky. Season with salt and freshly ground black pepper.

2. Bring a saucepan of salted water to the boil and cook the pasta for about 8 minutes, until al dente. Remove from the heat and plunge

the courgetti into the pan for 45 seconds to soften. Drain the pasta and leave in the sieve.

3. Transfer the pesto to the saucepan and heat gently. Add the pasta and courgetti, toss to coat thoroughly and serve immediately.

**Nutrition per serving:** 365 calories / 11.5g protein /4.5g fibre

## Crushed new potatoes with garlic and extra-virgin olive oil

With most fruits and veg, it's best not to peel them, as that is where the best nutrients are found. New potatoes are also to be less starchy than older ones and there is nothing like a garlicky crushed potato!

Serves 2

Prep time: 5 mins

Cook time 15 mins

300g new potatoes

20g butter

1 tsp grated garlic

5 sprigs of parsley, leaves picked and roughly chopped

Squeeze of fresh lemon juice

1. If some potatoes are bigger than others, cut the bigger ones in half to ensure even cooking.

2. Bring a saucepan of slightly salted water to the boil and add the potatoes. Return to the boil and cook for 10–15 minutes, or until tender. Drain and transfer to a serving bowl.

3. Place the butter and garlic in a small bowl and mash them together. Dot the garlic butter all over the potatoes and leave for a few moments to melt. Crush the potatoes with a potato masher, then season with salt and freshly ground black pepper. Scatter the parsley all over and finish with a squeeze of lemon juice.

**Nutrition per serving:** 185 calories / 3g protein / 3g fibre

# Parmesan roasted butternut squash

Roasted squash is irresistible and this recipe is so flexible – just mix up your cheese and other flavours.

Serves 2

Prep time: 5 mins

Cook time 20 mins

> 250g butternut squash (fresh or frozen), peeled and cut into chunks
> 1 tbsp olive oil
> 20g Parmesan, finely grated

1. Preheat the oven to 240°C/220°C Fan/Gas 9. Line a baking tray with parchment paper and place in the oven to get hot for 3 minutes.

2. Place the butternut squash in a bowl and break up any pieces that are stuck together. Toss with the olive oil, Parmesan and a pinch of salt and freshly ground black pepper.

3. Carefully remove the tray from the oven and scatter the butternut squash onto it in a single layer. Roast in the oven for 25–30 minutes, tossing halfway through.

**Nutrition per serving:** 142 calories / 5g protein / 3g fibre

# Crushed peas with lemon

Lightly crushed peas seem to have more flavour and are easier to eat! They are also one of the best plant-based sources of proteins, quick to cook, and easy to heat from frozen.

Serves 2
Prep time: 2 mins
Cook time 5 mins

> 200g frozen peas
> Zest of ½ lemon, plus 1 tsp juice
> A few sprigs of dill or parsley, finely chopped (optional)

1. Measure the peas into a small saucepan, cover with cold water and place over a high heat. Bring to the boil, remove from the heat and drain.

2. Transfer the peas to a serving bowl and toss with the lemon zest and juice. Scatter with the herbs, if using, and gently crush the peas. Season with salt and freshly ground black pepper to serve.

**Nutrition per serving**: 95 calories / 7g protein /5g fibre

# Kale and spinach with olives

Another delicious and versatile Mediterranean dish. Add a pinch of chilli flakes to give this side a warming kick.

Serves: 2

Prep time: 2 mins

Cook time: 4 mins

1 tbsp olive oil

100g kale, shredded

150g fresh spinach

10 pitted olives, roughly chopped (35g)

1. Place the olive oil in a large frying pan over a medium heat. When it is hot, add the kale and sauté for 2–3 minutes, or until wilted and softened.

2. Add the spinach and carefully mix with the kale. Cook for 1 minute, stirring all the time to help the leaves wilt evenly. Season with salt and freshly ground black pepper.

3. Transfer to a serving dish, top with the olives and serve.

**Nutrition per serving:** 116 calories / 4g protein / 5g fibre

# Sweet potato piri piri fries

Each different colour when you are 'eating the rainbow' provides important nutrients for health. These orange, fiery fries bring extra flavour, as well as feeding the gut microbiome.

Serves 2

Prep time: 5 mins

Cook time: 15 mins

> 1 large sweet potato, sliced lengthways into 1cm-wide fries
>     (350g prepared weight)
> 1 tbsp olive oil
> 1 tbsp piri piri seasoning

1. Preheat the oven to 240°C/220°C Fan/Gas 9. Line a large baking tray with parchment paper.

2. Place the sweet potato fries on the tray, drizzle with the olive oil and sprinkle with the piri piri seasoning. Season with salt and freshly ground black pepper and toss to coat.

3. Arrange the fries in a single layer, making sure they are not touching, and roast in the oven for 15 minutes, turning after 10 minutes.

**Nutrition per serving**: 236 calories / 2.5g protein / 6g fibre

## Raspberry yoghurt chocolate bites

Chocolate and raspberries are made for each other.

Makes 6

Prep time: 15 mins

100g raspberries
100g full-fat Greek yoghurt
1 tsp coconut oil
100g dark chocolate (70% cocoa solids), broken into small pieces

1. Line a baking tray with parchment paper.

2. Mix the raspberries with the yoghurt in a small bowl. Divide the mixture into 6 even spoonfuls and place on the baking tray. Transfer to the freezer for at least 30 minutes to set.

3. Melt the coconut oil and chocolate by placing them in a heatproof bowl over a pan of simmering water, or cooking in the microwave for 20 second intervals, stirring after each one.

4. Dip the frozen raspberry and yoghurt bites into the melted chocolate, making sure they are totally covered. The chocolate will set at once.

5. Store in the fridge for up to 3 hours, or keep them in the freezer. Allow them to soften for 30 minutes in the fridge before eating.

**Note**

These bites can be eaten straight from the freezer, if preferred.

**Nutrition per serving:** 119 calories / 2g protein / 1g fibre

# Chocolate-coated pistachio bites

Irresistible chocolate-coated pistachio bites with a creamy, nutty centre. These shouldn't spike your sugars.

Makes 16
Prep time: 10 mins

235ml coconut cream
120g pistachios, shelled (plus more to decorate)
8 pitted dates, diced
2 tsp vanilla extract
½ tsp ground cinnamon
Pinch of flaked sea salt
180g dark chocolate (70% cocoa solids), broken into pieces

1. Line a baking tray with parchment paper.

2. Blitz all ingredients, except the chocolate, together in a food processor or using a hand-held stick blender, leaving some texture.

3. Roll the mixture into balls the size of a grape, then place them on the prepared tray. Transfer to the fridge or freezer to firm up for about 1 hour.

4. Melt the chocolate in a heatproof bowl set over a pan of simmering water, or in the microwave.

5. Dip the pistachio balls in the chocolate to coat.

6. Store in the fridge for up to 3 hours, or keep them in the freezer. Allow them to soften for 30 minutes in the fridge before eating.

**Nutrition per serving:** 156 calories / 3g protein / 1g fibre

# Chocolate coconut cookies

You will love these little biscuits, made with no added sugar, and they shouldn't spike your blood sugars. As with most sweet treats, these are best eaten after a meal.

Serves 20
Prep time: 15 mins
Cook time: 15 mins

  60g coconut oil, plus ½ tsp melted

  120g ground almonds

  30g desiccated coconut

  1 large free-range egg

  ½ tsp baking powder

  1 tsp vanilla extract

  40g soft pitted dates, finely chopped

  40g dark chocolate chips (70% cocoa solids)

1. Preheat the oven to 180°C/160°C Fan/Gas 4. Grease a large baking tray with ½ teaspoon melted coconut oil.

2. Place all the remaining ingredients, except the chocolate, in a medium bowl. Add a generous pinch of salt and blitz briefly with a hand-held stick blender or in a food processor to make a slightly sticky mixture. You may need to add ½ tablespoon water if the mixture is a bit crumbly. Alternatively, mix together by hand.

3. Stir in the chocolate chips until well combined.

4. Roll the mixture into 20 small balls and place them on the greased tray. Flatten each one until around 1cm thick, then bake for about 15 minutes, or until firm and turning deep golden brown around the edges.

5. Leave to cool on the tray for a few minutes, then transfer to a wire rack. These store well in an airtight container in the freezer for up to 3 months.

**Nutrition per cookie:** 96 calories / 2g protein / 0.5g fibre

# Fruity pistachio bars

Gluten and dairy free, these indulgent fruity bars are easy to make and are portable, so you won't find yourself reaching for something that will send your sugars soaring!

Makes 12

Prep time: 6 mins

Cook time: 25 mins

80g pitted dates, diced

Grated zest and juice of 1 orange

80g dried apricots, diced

75g coconut oil

160g pistachios

Seeds from 2 cardamom pods (optional)

2 tbsp ground linseed

½ tsp salt

1. Preheat the oven to 180°C/160°C Fan/Gas 4. Line a 20cm square tin with parchment paper.

2. Soften the dates by heating them gently in the orange zest and juice in a small saucepan for 2 minutes.

3. Remove the pan from the heat and add the apricots and coconut oil. Set aside.

4. Blitz the pistachios and cardamom seeds (if using) with a hand-held stick blender or food processor to a coarse crumb. Add the date

and apricot mixture, the ground linseed and salt to the pistachios and blitz again.

5. Spoon the mixture into the tin, spreading it to the edges. Bake for 20–25 minutes, until just starting to brown a little on top. Remove from the oven and leave to cool slightly in the tin before cutting into 12 bars. Store in an airtight container for up to 5 days, or keep in the freezer for up to 3 months.

**Nutrition per serving:** 168 calories / 4g protein / 1.5g fibre

# Healthy gut black bean brownie

These brownies are super easy to make in one bowl. With gooey chocolate in the centre, they are very healthy and contain lots of fibre. Challenge anyone to guess the main ingredient!

Makes 12

Prep time: 8 mins

Cook times: 20 mins

1 × 400g tin black beans, drained and rinsed

3 medium free-range eggs

100g soft pitted dates

3 tbsp unsweetened cocoa powder

3 tbsp coconut oil

2 tsp vanilla extract

2 tbsp honey

30g dark chocolate chips (70% cocoa solids)

1. Preheat the oven to 190°C/170°C Fan/Gas 5. Line a 20cm square cake tin with parchment paper.

2. Place the black beans, eggs, dates, cocoa powder, coconut oil, vanilla extract, the honey and a pinch of salt in a food processor or blender. Blitz for about 2 minutes until really smooth.

3. Stir in the chocolate chips and pour the mixture into the prepared tin. Bake in the oven for 20 minutes.

4. Leave to cool in the tin, then slice into 12 squares to serve.

## Tip

Scatter with nuts of your choice for extra fibre and protein.

**Nutrition per brownie:** 115 calories / 4.5g protein / 3g fibre

# Savoury nuts

Michael was a fan of flavoured nuts to fill a little gap when he was hungry – they are well known for their health benefits and steady release of energy, and keep you full for longer, thanks to the fibre and protein. They also have anti-inflammatory properties, bolstering your immune system, as well as providing important nutrients, such as selenium, and can even provide protection from heart disease and type 2 diabetes.

Serves 4

Prep time: 5 mins

Cook time: 10 mins

- 120g mixed nuts (or nuts of your choice), any larger nuts roughly chopped
- 2 tsp melted coconut oil
- 1 tsp medium curry powder
- ½ tsp flaked sea salt
- ½ tsp dried chilli flakes (optional)

1. Preheat the oven to 180°C/160°C Fan/Gas 4.

2. Place the nuts in a medium bowl. Add all the remaining ingredients and lots of ground black pepper. Toss everything together until the nuts are lightly coated. Scatter over a baking tray and roast for 5 minutes.

3. Remove from the oven and turn the nuts. Roast for a further 5 minutes, or until the nuts are lightly browned. Take care they don't burn.

4. Cool for a few minutes on the tray to allow to crisp a little, then transfer to a bowl. Serve slightly warm or leave to cool completely.

**Nutrition per serving:** 193 calories / 8g protein / 0.5g fibre

# High-fibre peppery crackers

These savoury seeded crackers are very moreish, but they won't send sugars soaring. And with all that fabulous fibre, they will keep things moving, and those lovely microbes in your gut will love them too! These tasty crackers are perfect for dips, to scatter on a salad or soup. They also help top up your protein, too.

Makes 12

Prep time: 20 mins

Cook time: 30 mins

  3 tbsp wholegrain flour (or buckwheat)

  275g mixed seeds

  2 tbsp chia seeds

  ½–1 tsp freshly ground black pepper

  1–2 tsp flaked sea salt

1. Preheat the oven to 180°C/160°C Fan/Gas 4. Line a 33 × 23cm baking tray with parchment paper.

2. Mix all the ingredients in a medium bowl.

3. Pour in 200ml water and mix well. Leave to settle for about 15 minutes; the mixture will thicken and feel tacky.

4. Tip the dough on to the prepared baking tray and use a spatula to spread it out in a thin, even layer. Score it lightly, ready to separate into about 12 crackers. Bake for 15–20 minutes, until starting to

turn golden in places, then turn the crackers over and cook for about 15 minutes more. Don't overcook them or they will taste bitter. Turn off the oven and leave them to dry out in the oven for 1–2 hours.

5. Once cool, store in a sealed container for up to 1 week.

**Note**

If they become soft, you can pop them in the oven for 5 minutes to crisp up.

**Nutrition per serving**: 154 calories / 5.5g protein / 3g fibre

# Seeded nut loaf

This delicious, full-of-goodness loaf is packed with much-needed protein and fibre, and will keep for up to a week.

Makes: 1 loaf (12 slices)
Prep time: 7 mins
Cook time: 35 mins

40g pumpkin seeds
40g sunflower seeds
75g pistachios
50g poppy seeds
2 tbsp chia seeds
½ tbsp sea salt
3 medium free-range eggs
1 tbsp olive oil

1. Preheat the oven to 200°C/180°C Fan/Gas 6. Line a 450g loaf tin with parchment paper.

2. Place the pumpkin seeds, sunflower seeds, pistachios, poppy seeds and chia seeds in a bowl with the salt and mix together.

3. In a separate bowl whisk the eggs with the olive oil. Pour the egg mixture into the nuts and mix until thoroughly combined. Tip into the prepared tin and bake for 40 minutes. Leave to cool completely in the tin before slicing.

**Nutrition per slice:** 110 calories / 6g protein / 1g fibre

# Simple sauerkraut with coriander seeds

This is a classic sauerkraut, which provides plenty of flavour but adds minimal calories. We love the hint of coriander seeds, but feel free to experiment with other seeds, such as cumin, toasted coriander or mustard. Add to dishes for extra flavour, as you would a pickle.

Makes: 2 × 250ml jars

Prep time: 2 hours 15 mins, plus 1–2 weeks fermenting

½ medium red cabbage, quartered lengthwise, hard core removed, finely sliced

1½ red onions, halved and sliced

1 tsp coriander seeds

½ tbsp sea salt or kosher salt

2 × 250ml clean jam jars with tight-fitting lids

1. Mix the cabbage, onion and coriander seeds together in a large bowl, sprinkling the salt between the layers as you fill it. Massage the salt into the veg. Leave for 1–2 hours.

2. Spoon the cabbage mixture and juices into the jars.

3. Pack the mixture down in the jars, pressing it into the juices. Leave 1.5–2cm space at the top of each jar. If there is not enough liquid to cover the mixture, you can top up with either a few teaspoonfuls of filtered water or brine (1 teaspoon sea salt dissolved in 200ml filtered water).

4. Use a stone or piece of ceramic to keep the veg submerged, then seal the jars. Place the jars on a plate to catch any overflow and keep them at room temperature, out of direct sunlight. For the first few days, open the jars daily and press down the contents, to release the bubbles formed by the sauerkraut. Repeat this process every few days for 1–2 weeks (usually about one will do), until it is fermented to your taste.

5. The jars can be stored in the fridge for up to 2–3 months.

**Nutrition per 25g serving:** 8 calories / 0.5g protein / 1g fibre

# Mild, kimchi-style sauerkraut

Otherwise known as Asian sauerkraut, this spicy, exotic, strongly flavoured fermented vegetable dish is the core of Korean cuisine. This recipe is a milder version. We love having a spoonful for breakfast with an omelette or scrambled eggs.

Makes: 2 × 250ml jars

Prep time: 2 hours 15 mins, plus 1–2 weeks fermenting

- ½ medium white cabbage, quartered lengthwise, hard core removed, finely sliced
- 1½ red onions, halved and sliced
- ½ tbsp sea salt or kosher salt
- 2 tsp grated garlic
- 1 tsp grated fresh root ginger
- 1 tsp caster sugar
- 1 tbsp fish or soy sauce
- 2–4 tsp dried chilli flakes, according to taste
- 1 tsp sweet paprika
- 2 × 250ml clean jam jars with tight-fitting lids

1. Slice the cabbage into 1.5–2cm-wide ribbons. As with sauerkraut, mix it with the onion in a large bowl, sprinkling the salt between the layers as you fill it. Massage the salt into the veg. Leave it for about 2 hours.

2. Stir in the garlic and ginger and mix well.

3. Follow steps 2–5 of the sauerkraut recipe (pages 247–8) but add the extra step below.

4. After 3–4 days, gently mix in the rest of the ingredients (the cabbage won't ferment as effectively once the spices are included, so these need to be added a bit later in the process).

**Nutrition per 25g serving**: 10 calories / 0.5g protein / 1g fibre

# PART 5

# 7-DAY MEAL PLANNER

## 7-DAY MEAL PLANNER

| Day | |
|---|---|
| 1 | Mango and lime chia pots (page 169) |
| | Quick spinach and pea soup (pages 181–2) |
| | Roasted salmon and courgettes with anchovy chilli butter (pages 201–2) |
| 2 | Scrambled egg, Marmite and sourdough (page 180) |
| | Courgette and carrot fritters with coriander (pages 191–2) |
| | Smoked salmon, dill and caper pasta (pages 221–2) |
| 3 | Baked eggs with feta and spinach (page 176) |
| | Crunchy chicken salad with blue cheese dressing (page 189) |
| | Black pepper beef and veg stir fry (pages 219–20) |
| 4 | Cherry tomato and haricot bean bake (page 178) |
| | Greek spinach and feta pie (pages 193–4) |
| | One pot chicken with chickpeas, garlic and thyme (pages 203–4) |
| 5 | Green shakshuka (pages 171–2) |
| | Simple chowder (pages 183–4) |
| | Black bean chilli with butternut squash and spinach (pages 199–200) |
| 6 | Salmon and rocket egg muffins (page 173) |
| | Mackerel and beetroot salad (page 186) |
| | Trapanese courgetti pasta (pages 223–4) |
| 7 | Mushrooms on toast (page 179) |
| | Smashed chilli avocado with fried egg and sauerkraut (page 185) |
| | Gut-friendly shepherd's pie (pages 209–10) |

| | Calories (kcal) | Protein (g) | Fibre (g) |
|---|---|---|---|
| | 174 | 9 | 6.5 |
| | 204 | 9 | 9 |
| | 501 | 30.5 | 3.5 |
| | 215 | 13 | 3 |
| | 309 | 17 | 3.5 |
| | 359 | 19 | 6 |
| | 260 | 23 | 3 |
| | 308 | 30 | 2 |
| | 332 | 31 | 5.5 |
| | 189 | 5 | 6 |
| | 194 | 7 | 3 |
| | 510 | 54 | 8 |
| | 310 | 13 | 4.5 |
| | 232 | 25 | 3 |
| | 292 | 14.5 | 19.5 |
| | 90 | 5.5 | 0 |
| | 442 | 25 | 3 |
| | 365 | 11.5 | 4.5 |
| | 272 | 5.5 | 3 |
| | 324 | 13 | 6 |
| | 400 | 22.5 | 8 |

# CONVERSION TABLES

## Weight

5g ............... ⅛oz
10g ........... ¼oz
15g ........... ½oz
20g ........... ¾oz
25/30g .... 1oz
35g ........... 1¼oz
40/45g ..... 1½oz
50g ........... 1¾oz
60g ........... 2¼oz
70g ........... 2½oz
75g ........... 2⅔oz
80g ........... 2¾oz
90g ........... 3¼oz
100g ........ 3½oz
115g ......... 4oz
120g ........ 4¼oz
125g ......... 4½oz
150g ........ 5⅓oz
160g ........ 5⅔oz
180g ......... 6¼oz
200g ........ 7oz
240g ........ 8½oz
250g ......... 9oz
275g ......... 9⅓oz
280g ........ 9¾oz
300g ........ 10½oz
340g ........ 12oz
350g ......... 12⅓oz
375g .......... 13oz
400g ........ 14oz
450g ......... 1lb
500g ........ 1lb 2oz

## Volume

30ml ............. 1fl oz
50ml ............. 1¾fl oz
75ml ............. 2⅔fl oz
85ml ............. 3fl oz
100ml ......... 3½fl oz
120ml ........... 4¼fl oz
125ml ........... 4⅓fl oz
150ml ......... 5¼fl oz (¼ pint)
175ml .......... 6fl oz
200ml ......... 7fl oz (⅓ pint)
225ml ........... 8fl oz
235ml ........... 8¼fl oz
240ml ........... 8½fl oz
250ml ........... 8¾fl oz
270ml ........... 9½fl oz
300ml ......... 10½fl oz (½ pint)
350ml ........... 12⅓fl oz
400ml ......... 14fl oz
450ml ........... 15¾fl oz (¾ pint)
500ml ......... 17⅔fl oz
600ml ......... 21fl oz (1 pint)
700ml ............ 24½fl oz (1¼ pint)
800ml ......... 28fl oz

## Measurements

1cm ............... ½in
1.5cm ........... ⅔in
2cm ............... ¾in
2.5cm .......... 1in
5cm ............... 2in
10cm ............. 4in
11cm ............. 4¼in
12cm ............ 4½in
12.5cm ......... 5in
13cm ............ 5¼in
14cm ............. 5½in
15cm ............. 6in
16cm ............. 6¼in
17cm ............. 6½in
18cm ............. 7in
19cm ............. 7½in
20cm ............. 8in
21cm ............. 8¼in
22cm ............. 8½in
23cm ............. 9in
24cm ............. 9½in
25cm ............. 10in
26cm ............. 10½in
27cm ............. 10¾in
28cm ............. 11in
29cm ............. 11½in
30cm ............. 12in
31cm ............. 12½in
32cm ............. 12¾in
33cm ............. 13in

# UK/US TERMS

| UK | US |
|---|---|
| Aubergine | Eggplant |
| Baby gem lettuce | Little gem lettuce |
| Baking paper | Parchment paper |
| Baking tray | Baking sheet |
| Beetroot | Beets |
| Cannellini beans | White kidney beans |
| Caster sugar | Superfine sugar |
| Chickpeas | Garbanzo beans |
| Coriander (fresh) | Cilantro |
| Courgette | Zucchini |
| Dark chocolate | Semi-sweet chocolate |
| Dried chilli flakes | Red pepper flakes |
| Filo pastry | Phyllo pastry |
| Frying pan | Skillet |
| Full-fat milk | Whole milk |
| Grill | Broiler |
| Haricot beans | Navy beans |
| Linseed | Flaxseed |
| Marmite | Yeast extract |
| Minced beef | Ground beef |
| Pak choi | Bok choy |
| Pepper | Bell pepper |
| Prawn | Shrimp |
| Puy lentils | French green lentils |
| Rocket | Arugula |
| Sieve | Strainer |
| Stock cube | Bouillon cube |
| Tin | Pan |
| Whisk | Beat |
| Wholegrain/wholemeal | Wholewheat |
| Zest | Rind |

# ACKNOWLEDGEMENTS

It has been a tough six months for the family and me. I couldn't have got through it without their support. One positive to come from it all is that we have become closer as a family, which Dad would have loved to see.

I would like to thank my mum first all of, who has been so incredibly strong through such a difficult time. She has also provided help and guidance for me while writing this book, as well as providing excellent recipes with her own special touch! I'd like to thank my amazing fiancée, Heather, who has been an incredible rock over the last six months, from start to finish, from leaving for Symi and everything in between. Without her encouragement, I doubt I would have finished this book.

Thank you to my siblings, Alex, Dan and Kate, and their wonderful partners. They have provided fantastic advice and assistance during the writing process.

Thanks to my in-laws, Martin and Sue, who have provided a great deal of support and advice along the way.

A big thank you to Louise Atkinson, my brilliant editor, who was crucial to the writing of the book! Also huge thanks to the brilliant food writer Kathryn Bruton, who works alongside my mum, as well as Jo Roberts-Miller, the super-efficient copyeditor.

Thank you to my wonderful agent, Sophie Laurimore, and also Zoë Parrish at the SOHO agency.

Thank you to all those at Octopus publishing, including Jo Morrell, Katie Forsythe, Leanne Bryan and everyone behind the scenes, who believed in the book and helped make it happen.

Thank you to all of those who took time out of their day to provide fantastic interviews for me: Professor Felice Jacka, Professor Roy Taylor, Dr Patrick Garratt, Dr David Unwin, Dr Tanya Smith, Dr Pawel, Adele, Elisette, Peter, Simon and those I spoke to who wish to remain anonymous!

And, of course, thank you to my dad for everything you have done for us. You provided the inspiration to write this book in the first place. You will be greatly missed.

# ENDNOTES

## Chapter 1: The Rise of Obesity

1.  O'Hare, R. (2024) 'More than one billion people now living with obesity, global analysis suggests', Imperial News, Imperial College London. Available at: https://www.imperial. ac.uk/news/251798/more-than-billion-people-living-with/#:~:text=From%20 1990%20to%202022%2C%20global,from%2016.7%25%20to%2010.8%25.

2.  Office for Health Improvement and Disparities (2024) 'Obesity profile: short statistical commentary'. Available at: https://www.gov.uk/government/statistics/update-to-the-obesity-profile-on-fingertips/obesity-profile-short-statistical-commentary-may-2024

3.  Centers for Disease Control and Prevention (CDC) (2024) 'Adult obesity facts'. Available at: https://www.cdc.gov/obesity/adult-obesity-facts/

4.  Kyrou, I., Randeva, H.S., Tsigos, H.H., *et al*. (2018) 'Clinical problems caused by obesity'. Available at: https://europepmc.org/article/MED/25905207/NBK278943#free-full-text

5.  Seino, Y., Fukushima, M. and Yabe, D. (2010) 'GIP and GLP-1, the two incretin hormones: similarities and differences', *Journal of Diabetes Investigation*, 22;1(1–2):8–23. doi: 10.1111/j.2040–1124.2010.00022.x. Available at: https://pmc.ncbi.nlm.nih. gov/articles/PMC4020673/

6.  Cancer Research UK (2023) 'How does obesity cause cancer?'. Available at: https:// www.cancerresearchuk.org/about-cancer/causes-of-cancer/bodyweight-and-cancer/ how-does-obesity-cause-cancer

7.  Deshpande, A.D., Harris-Hayes, M., and M. Schootman, *Epidemiology of Diabetes and Diabetes-Related Complications*, American Physical Therapy Association 2008: p. 125–164. Available at: https://pubmed.ncbi.nlm.nih.gov/18801858/

    Public Health England (2014) Adult obesity and type 2 diabetes. Available at: chrome-extension://efaidnbmnnnibpcajpcglclefindmkaj/https://assets.publishing.service.gov. uk/media/5a7f069140f0b6230268d059/Adult_obesity_and_type_2_diabetes_.pdf

8.  Food, Farming and Countryside Commission (2024) 'Unhealthy food costing UK billions'. Available at: https://ffcc.co.uk/news-and-press/unhealthy-food-costing-uk-billions

#:~:text=New%20analysis%20commissioned%20by%20the,total%20annual%20
UK%20healthcare%20spend

9. Frijters, P., Clark, A.E., Krekel, C. and Layard, R. (2020) 'A happy choice: wellbeing as the goal of government', *Behavioural Public Policy*. Available at: https://www.cambridge. org/core/journals/behavioural-public-policy/article/abs/happy-choice-wellbeing-as-the-goal-of-government/ED3A4E384D726238CC2524932F868CBD

10. McKinsey Health Institute (2022) *Adding years to life and life to years*. Available at: https://www.mckinsey.com/mhi/our-insights/adding-years-to-life-and-life-to-years# section-header-1

11. Change 4 Life (n.d.) 'Slimming 60s to baby boomers booming'. Available at: chrome-extension://efaidnbmnnnibpcajpcglclefindmkaj/https://fullfact.org/sites/fullfact.org/ files/2012/06/Slimming_60s_to_Baby_Boomers_Booming_FINAL.pdf

12. Kim, S.Y., and Yi, D.Y. (2020) 'Components of human breast milk: from macronutrient to microbiome and microRNA', *Clinical and Experimental Pediatrics*, 23;63(8):301– 309. doi: 10.3345/cep.2020.00059. Available at: https://pmc.ncbi.nlm.nih.gov/articles/ PMC7402982/

13. BBC Food (2024) 'What's the right portion size for you?'. Available at: https://www.bbc. co.uk/food/articles/portion_size

14. Rhonda, S., Sebastian, M.A., Wilkinson Enns, C., and Goldman, J.D. (2011) 'Snacking patterns of U.S. adults'. Food Surveys Research Group. Available at: chrome-extension://efaidnbmnnnibpcajpcglclefindmkaj/https://www.ars.usda.gov/ ARSUserFiles/80400530/pdf/dbrief/4_adult_snacking_0708.pdf

Food Surveys Research Group (2020) 'Snack Consumption by U.S. Adults: What We Eat in America. NHANES 2017 – March 2020'. Available at: chrome-extension:// efaidnbmnnnibpcajpcglclefindmkaj/https://www.ars.usda.gov/ARSUserFiles/ 80400530/pdf/DBrief/53_Snacks_Consumption_by_Adults_1720.pdf

15. Taylor, R., Barnes, A.C., Hollingsworth, K.G., *et al*. (2023) 'Aetiology of Type 2 diabetes in people with a 'normal' body mass index: testing the personal fat threshold hypothesis', Clin Sci, 31;137(16):1333–1346. doi: 10.1042/CS20230586. Available at: https:// pmc.ncbi.nlm.nih.gov/articles/PMC10472166/#:~:text=The%20Personal%20 Fat%20Threshold%20hypothesis%20postulates%20that%20people%20with%20 T2D,glucose%20control%20after%20weight%20loss.

16. Taylor, R. (20) 'Banting Memorial Lecture 2012 Reversing the twin cycles of Type2 diabetes', *Diabetic* Medicine, DOI:10.1111/dme.12039. Available at:

chrome-extension://efaidnbmnnnibpcajpcglclefindmkaj/https://www.ncl.ac.uk/media/wwwnclacuk/newcastlemagneticresonancecentre/files/banting-memorial-lecture.pdf

17. Mittal, B. (2019) 'Subcutaneous adipose tissue & visceral adipose tissue', *Indian Journal of Medical Research*, 149(5):571–573. doi: 10.4103/ijmr.IJMR_1910_18. Available at: https://pmc.ncbi.nlm.nih.gov/articles/PMC6702693/

18. Ryan, D.H., and Yocket, S.R. (2017) 'Weight loss and improvement in comorbidity: differences at 5%, 10%, 15%, and over', Curr Obes Rep., 6(2):187–194. doi: 10.1007/s13679-017-0262-y. Available at: https://pubmed.ncbi.nlm.nih.gov/28455679/

19. Magkos, F., Fraterrigo, G., Yoshino, J., *et al.* (2016) 'Effects of moderate and subsequent progressive weight loss on metabolic function and adipose tissue biology in humans with obesity', *Cell Metab.*, 23(4):591–601. doi: 10.1016/j.cmet.2016.02.005. Available at: https://pubmed.ncbi.nlm.nih.gov/26916363/

## Chapter 2: A Paradox – Overfed Yet Undernourished

1. Bradley, M., Melchor, J., Carr, R., and Karjoo, S. (2023) 'Obesity and malnutrition in children and adults: a clinical review', *Obesity Pillars,* 8. Available at: https://www.sciencedirect.com/science/article/pii/S2667368123000335#bib5

2. Soysal, P., Koc Okudur, S., Kilic, N., *et al.* (2022) 'The prevalence of undernutrition and associated factors in older obese patients', *Aging Clin Exp Res.*, 34(9):2023–2030. doi: 10.1007/s40520-022-02143-7. Available at: https://pubmed.ncbi.nlm.nih.gov/35575948/#:~:text=Those%20who%20were%20not%20well,%C2%A9%202022.

3. Price, C. (2017) 'The age of scurvy', *Distillations Magazine*, Science History Institute. Available at: https://www.sciencehistory.org/stories/magazine/the-age-of-scurvy/#:~:text=Scurvy per cent20killed per cent20more per cent20than per cent20two,determining per cent20the per cent20destiny per cent20of per cent20nations. per centE2 per cent80 per cent9D

4. ABC News (2024) 'Doctors discover case of scurvy in Western Australia, warn it is a "re-emerging diagnosis"'. Available at: https://www.abc.net.au/news/2024-10-23/scurvy-case-detected-western-australia/104503318

5. Morris, S. (2016) 'Boy who died of scurvy "invisible" to authorities, says leaked report', *Guardian*, 22 January. Available at: https://www.theguardian.com/society/2016/jan/22/concerns-raised-about-boy-who-died-of-scurvy-a-year-before-his-death-leaked-report

Lambert, G. (2023) 'Thousands of people admitted to hospital with malnutrition'. *The Times*. 10 July. Available at: https://www.thetimes.com/article/times-health-commission-thousands-of-people-admitted-to-hospital-suffering-from-malnutrition-n23hqgzjr

6. Dighe, S., Zhao, J., Steffen, L., *et al.* (2020) 'Diet patterns and the incidence of age-related macular degeneration in the Atherosclerosis Risk in Communities (ARIC) study', *British Journal of Ophthalmology*,104:1070–1076. Available at: https://bjo.bmj.com/content/104/8/1070

7. BBC News (2013) 'Men's average height up 11cm since 1870s'. Available at: https://www.bbc.co.uk/news/health-23896855

8. House of Lords Food, Diet and Obesity Committee (2024) 'We need a plan to fix our broken food system'. Available at: https://ukparliament.shorthandstories.com/food-diet-obesity-lords-report/index.html?utm_source=committees.parliament.uk&utm_medium=referral+&utm_campaign=food-diet-obesity-report&utm_content=launch-news-story

9. The Food Foundation (2024) 'Health and food experts warning amid significant decline in children's health', press release, 19 June. Available at: https://foodfoundation.org.uk/press-release/health-and-food-experts-warning-amid-significant-decline-childrens-health#:~:text=Health%20and%20food%20experts%20warning%20amid%20significant%20decline%20in%20children%27s%20health,-%EF%82%9A%20%EF%82%99%20%EF%83%A0&text=Health%20and%20food%20experts%20and,babies%20born%20a%20decade%20ago

10. Lambert, G. (2023) 'Thousands of people admitted to hospital with malnutrition', *The Times*,10 July. Available at: https://www.thetimes.com/article/times-health-commission-thousands-of-people-admitted-to-hospital-suffering-from-malnutrition-n23hqgzjr

11. Martini, D., Godos, J., Bonaccio, M., *et al.* (2021) 'Ultra-processed foods and nutritional dietary profile: a meta-analysis of nationally representative samples', *Nutrients*, 13(10):3390. doi: 10.3390/nu13103390. Available at: https://pmc.ncbi.nlm.nih.gov/articles/PMC8538030/#sec2-nutrients-13-03390

12. Piuri, G., Zocchi, M., Della Porta, M., *et al.* (2021) 'Magnesium in obesity, metabolic syndrome, and type 2 diabetes', *Nutrients*, *13*(2): 320 Available at: https://www.mdpi.com/2072-6643/13/2/320.

Razzaque, M.S. (2018) 'Magnesium: are we consuming enough?', *Nutrients,* 10(12): 1863. doi: 10.3390/nu10121863. Available at: https://pmc.ncbi.nlm.nih.gov/articles/PMC6316205/

13. NHS England Digital (2020) 'Scurvy, rickets and malnutrition admissions, by age, 2007–08 to 2019–20'. Available at: https://digital.nhs.uk/supplementary-information/2020/scurvy-rickets-and-malnutrition-admissions-by-age-2007-08-to-2019-20

14. Lange, J. and Königsrainer, A. (2019) 'Malnutrition as a complication of bariatric surgery – a clear and present danger?', *Visceral Medicine*, 35(5):305–311. doi: 10.1159/000503040. Available at: https://pmc.ncbi.nlm.nih.gov/articles/PMC6873028/

## Chapter 3: Muscle Loss

1. Volpi, E., Nazemi, R. and Fujita, S. (2004) 'Muscle tissue changes with aging', *Curr Opin Clin Nutr Metab Care,* 7(4):405-10. doi: 10.1097/01.mco.0000134362.76653.b2. Available at: https://pmc.ncbi.nlm.nih.gov/articles/PMC2804956/#:~:text=Introduction,%2C%20heart%20disease%2C%20and%20osteoporosis.

2. Merz, K.E., and Thurmond, D.C. (2020) 'Role of skeletal muscle in insulin resistance and glucose uptake', *Compr Physiol.*, 10(3):785–809. doi: 10.1002/cphy.c190029. Available at: https://pmc.ncbi.nlm.nih.gov/articles/PMC8074531/

3. Musalek, C. and Kirchengast, S. (2017) 'Grip strength as an indicator of health-related quality of life in old age-a pilot study', *Int J Environ Res Public Health*, 14(12):1447. doi: 10.3390/ijerph14121447. Available at: https://pmc.ncbi.nlm.nih.gov/articles/PMC5750866/

    Syddall, H.E., Westbury, L.D., Shaw, S.C., *et al.* (2018) 'Correlates of level and loss of grip strength in later life: findings from the English Longitudinal Study of Ageing and the Hertfordshire Cohort Study', *Calcif Tissue Int*, 102, 53–63. https://doi.org/10.1007/s00223-017-0337-5. Available at: https://link.springer.com/article/10.1007/s00223-017-0337-5#citeas

4. Syddall, H., Cooper, C., Martin, F. (2003) 'Is grip strength a useful single marker of frailty?', *Age and Ageing*, 32(6): 650–656, https://doi.org/10.1093/ageing/afg111. Available at: https://academic.oup.com/ageing/article-abstract/32/6/650/13078?redirectedFrom=fulltext

    Leong, D.P., Teo, K.K., Rangarajan, S., *et al.*, (2015) 'Prognostic value of grip strength: findings from the Prospective Urban Rural Epidemiology (PURE) study',

*The Lancet*, 386(9990): 266 – 273. Available at: https://www.thelancet.com/journals/lancet/article/PIIS0140-6736(14)62000-6/abstract

5.  Yang, N.P., Hsu, N.W., Lin, C.H., *et al.* (2018) 'Relationship between muscle strength and fall episodes among the elderly: the Yilan study, Taiwan', *BMC Geriatr*, 18, 90. https://doi.org/10.1186/s12877-018-0779-2 Available at: https://bmcgeriatr. biomedcentral.com/articles/10.1186/s12877-018-0779-2#citeas

6.  Cava, E., Yeat, N.C., and Mittendorfer, B. (2017) 'Preserving healthy muscle during weight loss', *Adv Nutr.*, 8(3):511–519. doi: 10.3945/an.116.014506. Available at: https:// pmc.ncbi.nlm.nih.gov/articles/PMC5421125/

7.  Wilding, J.P.H., Batterham, R.L., Calanna, S., *et al.* (2021) 'Once-weekly semaglutide in adults with overweight or obesity', *New England Journal of Medicine,* Supplement 384:989–1002. DOI: 10.1056/NEJMoa2032183. Available at: nejmoa2032183_appendix.pdf

8.  Wilding, J.P.H., Batterham, R.L., Davies, M., *et al.* (2022) 'Weight regain and cardiometabolic effects after withdrawal of semaglutide: the STEP 1 trial extension'. *Diabetes, Obesity and Metabolism,* 24(8); 1553–64. Available at: chrome-extension:// efaidnbmnnnibpcajpcglclefindmkaj/https://discovery.ucl.ac.uk/id/eprint/10149199/1/ Diabetes%20Obesity%20Metabolism%20-%202022%20-%20Wilding% 20-%20Weight%20regain%20and%20cardiometabolic%20effects%20after%20 withdrawal%20of%20semaglutide%20.pdf

9.  Epocrates (2024) 'Obesity drugs' success spurs rush in muscle-preserving drug research'. Available at: https://www.epocrates.com/online/article/obesity-drugs-success-spurs-rush-in-muscle-preserving-drug-research

10. Heymsfield, S.B., Coleman, L.A., Miller, R., *et al.* (2021) 'Effect of Bimagrumab vs placebo on body fat mass among adults with type 2 diabetes and obesity: a phase 2 randomized clinical trial', *JAMA Netw Open*, 4(1):e2033457. doi:10.1001/ jamanetworkopen.2020.33457. Available at: https://jamanetwork.com/journals/ jamanetworkopen/fullarticle/2774903

11. Beavers, K.M., Lyles, M.F., Davis Cralen, C., *et al.* (2011) 'Is lost lean mass from intentional weight loss recovered during weight regain in postmenopausal women?', *American Journal of Clinical Nutrition*, 94(3); 767–774. Available at: https://www. sciencedirect.com/science/article/pii/S0002916523024322

12. Yates, T., Biddle, G.J.H., Henson, J., *et al.* (2023) 'Impact of weight loss and weight gain trajectories on body composition in a population at high risk of type 2 diabetes:

a prospective cohort analysis', *Diabetes, Obesity and Metabolism*, 26(30): 1008–1015. Available at: https://dom-pubs.onlinelibrary.wiley.com/doi/10.1111/dom.15400

13. University of Leicester (2023) 'Weight re-gained after weight loss results in less muscle, more fat, study finds'. Available at: https://le.ac.uk/news/2023/december/overweight#:~:text= News-,Weight%20re%2Dgained%20after%20weight%20loss%20results%20 in,muscle%2C%20more%20fat%2C%20study%20finds&text=A%20Leicester%20 study%20that%20measured,negative%20impact%20on%20muscle%20mass.

14. National Institute of Aging (2022) 'How can strength training build healthier bodies as we age?'. Available at: https://www.nia.nih.gov/news/how-can-strength-training-build-healthier-bodies-we-age

15. Villareal, D.T,. Aguirre, L., Gurney, A.B., (2017) 'Aerobic or resistance exercise, or both, in dieting obese older adults', *New England Journal of Medicine*, 376(20):1943–1955. doi: 10.1056/NEJMoa1616338. Available at: https://pubmed.ncbi.nlm.nih.gov/28514618/

   NBC News (2023) 'Weight loss drugs can lead to muscle loss, too. Is that a bad thing?'. Available at: https://www.nbcnews.com/health/health-news/weight-loss-drugs-muscle-loss-rcna84936

   BBC Future (2024) 'What happens when you stop taking weight-loss drugs?'. Available at: https://www.bbc.com/future/article/20240521-what-happens-when-you-stop-taking-ozempic

## Chapter 4: The Journey to Discovery

1. Garrow, J.S., and Gardiner, G.T. ( 1981) 'Maintenance of weight loss in obese patients after jaw wiring', *Br Med J (Clin Res Ed)*, 282(6267):858–60. doi: 10.1136/bmj.282.6267.858. Available at: https://www.ncbi.nlm.nih.gov/pmc/articles/PMC1504679

2. Cohen, A. (1998) 'Fen-phen and valvular heart disease'. *Nutrition Bytes*, 4(3). Available at: https://escholarship.org/uc/item/4vt2x92w

   SoRelle, R. (1999) 'Diet drug maker agrees to $3.75 billion settlement', *Circulation*, 100(25). Available at: https://www.ahajournals.org/doi/full/10.1161/01.CIR.100.25.e133.

3. Matei, D., Trofin, D., Iordan, D.A., *et al.* (2023) 'The endocannabinoid system and physical exercise', *Int J Mol Sci.*, 24(3):1989. doi: 10.3390/ijms24031989. Available at: https://pmc.ncbi.nlm.nih.gov/articles/PMC9916354/

   Topol, E.J., Bousser, M.G., Fox, K.A., *et al.* (2010) 'Rimonabant for prevention of cardiovascular events (CRESCENDO): a randomised, multicentre, placebo-controlled trial', *Lancet*, 14;376(9740):517–23. doi: 10.1016/S0140-6736(10)60935-X. Available at: https://pubmed.ncbi.nlm.nih.gov/20709233/

Bray, G.A., and Purnell, J.Q. (2022) 'An historical review of steps and missteps in the discovery of anti-obesity drugs' [updated 2022 Jul 10]. In: Feingold K R, Anawalt B, Blackman M.R., *et al.*, editors. Endotext [Internet]. South Dartmouth (MA). Available at: https://www.ncbi.nlm.nih.gov/books/NBK581942/

4. *Guardian* ( 2010) 'Anti-obesity drug Reductil banned across Europe', 22 January. Available at: https://www.theguardian.com/lifeandstyle/2010/jan/22/reductil-banned-in-europe

5. Maciejewski, M.L., Arterburn, D.E., Van Scoyoc, L., *et al.* (2016) 'Bariatric surgery and long-term durability of weight loss', *JAMA Surg.,* 151(11):1046–1055. doi:10.1001/jamasurg.2016.2317. Available at: https://jamanetwork.com/journals/jamasurgery/fullarticle/2546331

6. Poires, W. (2008) 'Bariatric surgery: risks and rewards', *The Journal of Clinical Endocrinology & Metabolism*, 93(11)S1: s89–s96, https://doi.org/10.1210/jc.2008-1641. Available at: https://academic.oup.com/jcem/article/93/11_supplement_1/s89/2627224

Chang, S., Stoll, C.R.T., Song, J., *et al.* (2014) 'The effectiveness and risks of bariatric surgery: an updated systematic review and meta-analysis, 2003–2012', *JAMA Surg.,* 149(3):275–287. doi:10.1001/jamasurg.2013.3654. Available at: https://jamanetwork.com/journals/jamasurgery/fullarticle/1790378/

7. Mojsov, S., Weir, G.C. and Habener, J.F. (1987) 'Insulinotropin: glucagon-like peptide I (7-37) co-encoded in the glucagon gene is a potent stimulator of insulin release in the perfused rat pancreas', *Journal of Clinical Investigation*, 79(2). Available at: https://www.jci.org/articles/view/112855

Drucker, D.J., Philippe, J., Mojsov, S., and Habener, J.F. (1987) 'Glucagon-like peptide I stimulates insulin gene expression and increases cyclic AMP levels in a rat islet cell line', *Proc Natl Acad Sci USA*, 84(10):3434–8. doi: 10.1073/pnas.84.10.3434. Available at: https://pmc.ncbi.nlm.nih.gov/articles/PMC304885/

8. National Institute of Aging (2012) 'Exendin-4: From lizard to laboratory . . .and beyond'. Available at: https://www.nia.nih.gov/news/exendin-4-lizard-laboratory-and-beyond

9. ScienceDirect (n.d.) 'Exendin-4 - an overview'. Available at: https://www.sciencedirect.com/topics/chemistry/exendin-4#:~:text=Furthermore per cent2C per cent20exendin per cent2D4 per cent20has per cent20longer,IV per cent20(DPP per cent2D1V).

Kolterman, O.G., Buse, J.B., Fineman, M.S., *et al.* (2003) 'Synthetic exendin-4 (exenatide) significantly reduces postprandial and fasting plasma glucose in subjects with type 2 diabetes', *J Clin Endocrinol Metab.*, 88(7):3082–9. doi: 10.1210/jc.2002-021545. Available at: https://pubmed.ncbi.nlm.nih.gov/12843147/

Los Angeles Zoo (n.d.) 'Gila monster'. Available at: https://lazoo.org/explore-your-zoo/our-animals/reptiles/gila-monster/#:~:text=In per cent20order per cent20to per cent20cope per cent20with,to per cent20avoid per cent20the per cent20harsh per cent20sun.

10. Eng, J., Knleinman, W.A., Singh, L., *et al.* (1992) 'Isolation and characterization of exendin-4, an exendin-3 analogue, from Heloderma suspectum venom. Further evidence for an exendin receptor on dispersed acini from guinea pig pancreas'. *Journal of Biological Chemistry*, 267(11): 7402–05. Available at: https://www.jbc.org/article/S0021-9258(18)42531-8/pdf

11. CDD Vault (2023) 'Drug Discovery Industry Roundup with Barry Bunin – August 30, 2023'. Available at: https://www.collaborativedrug.com/cdd-blog/drug-discovery-industry-roundup-barry-bunin-august-30-2023

*New York Times* (2023) 'Where Ozempic, Wegovy and New Weight Loss Drugs Came From', 17 August. Available at: https://www.nytimes.com/2023/08/17/health/weight-loss-drugs-obesity-ozempic-wegovy.html

12. *The Times* (2024) 'The lizard, the wonder drug – and how it will change the world', 17 May. Available at: https://www.thetimes.com/comment/columnists/article/the-lizard-the-wonder-drug-and-how-it-will-change-the-world-zjlxj6zc6

13. *Global News* (2023) 'How a Canadian scientist and a venomous lizard helped pave the way for Ozempic', 28 June. Available at: https://globalnews.ca/news/9793403/ozempic-canada-scientist-venomous-lizard-weight-loss/

Chen, Y.E. and Drucker, D.J. (1997) 'Tissue-specific Expression of Unique mRNAs That Encode Proglucagon-derived Peptides or Exendin 4 in the Lizard', *Journal of Biological Chemistry*, 272(7): 4108–4115. Available at: https://www.jbc.org/article/S0021-9258(19)67267-4/fulltext

Kolterman, O.G., O.G., Buse, J.B., Fineman, M.S., *et al.* (2003) 'Synthetic exendin-4 (exenatide) significantly reduces postprandial and fasting plasma glucose in subjects with type 2 diabetes', *J Clin Endocrinol Metab.,* 88(7):3082–9. doi: 10.1210/jc.2002-021545. Available at: https://pubmed.ncbi.nlm.nih.gov/12843147/

14. *New York Times* (2023) 'Where Ozempic, Wegovy and New Weight Loss Drugs Came From', 17 August. Available at: https://www.nytimes.com/2023/08/17/health/weight-loss-drugs-obesity-ozempic-wegovy.html

15. *Maclean's* (2024) 'The Canadian doctor who helped invent Ozempic'. Available at: https://macleans.ca/society/health/who-discovered-ozempic/

16. The free weekly newsletter 'Diabetes In Control' spoke to Eng back in 2007.

17. 'Diabetes Drug Byetta Gets FDA Approval'. Available at: https://www.wcgclinical.com/fdanews/

   *Diabetes in Control* (2007) 'Dr John Eng's Research Found That The Saliva Of The Gila Monster Contains A Hormone That Treats Diabetes Better Than Any Other Medicine'. Available at: https://www.diabetesincontrol.com/dr-john-engs-research-found-that-the-saliva-of-the-gila-monster-contains-a-hormone-that-treats-diabetes-better-than-any-other-medicine/

   National Institute on Aging (2012) 'Exendin-4: From lizard to laboratory...and beyond'. Available at: https://www.nia.nih.gov/news/exendin-4-lizard-laboratory-and-beyond

   *Maclean's* (2024) 'The Canadian doctor who helped invent Ozempic'. Available at: https://macleans.ca/society/health/who-discovered-ozempic/

18. Collins, L. and Costello, R.A. (2024) 'Glucagon-like peptide-1 receptor agonists', *StatPearls*. Available at: https://www.ncbi.nlm.nih.gov/books/NBK551568/

19. Dushay J., Gao, C., Gopalakrishnan, G.S., *et al*. (2012) 'Short-term exenatide treatment leads to significant weight loss in a subset of obese women without diabetes', *Diabetes Care,* 35(1):4–11. doi: 10.2337/dc11-0931. Available at: https://pmc.ncbi.nlm.nih.gov/articles/PMC3241299/

   US Food and Drug Administration (2020) 'Drug trial snapshot: Ozempic'. Available at: https://www.fda.gov/drugs/drug-approvals-and-databases/drug-trial-snapshot-ozempic

20. *Time* (2024) 'Ozempic gets the Oprah treatment in a new TV special'. Available at: https://time.com/6958224/oprah-weight-loss-special-ozempic/

21. *Times of India* (2024) 'Elon Musk looks fitter than ever: secrets behind his rapid and lasting weight loss'. Available at: https://timesofindia.indiatimes.com/life-style/health-fitness/weight-loss/elon-musk-looks-fitter-than-ever-secrets-behind-his-rapid-and-lasting-weight-loss/articleshow/116145248.cms

22. ABC News (2024) 'Elon Musk shows support for weight loss drugs despite RFK Jr.'s criticism'. Available at: https://abcnews.go.com/US/elon-musk-shows-support-weight-loss-drugs-despite/story?id=116706006

23. *CEO World Magazine* (20204) 'Europe's largest companies by market capitalization, 2024'. Available at: https://ceoworld.biz/2024/02/14/europes-largest-companies-by-market-capitalization-2024/#:~:text=As%20of%20September%2017%2C%20 2024,Holding%20NV%20(%24315%20billion).

24. Applied Clinical Trials (2023) 'FDA approves significant new treatment for chronic weight management '. Available at: https://www.appliedclinicaltrialsonline.com/view/fda-approves-significant-new-treatment-for-chronic-weight-management

      Jastreboff, A.M., Aronne, L.J., Ahmad, N.N., *et al.* (2022) 'Tirzepatide once weekly for the treatment of obesity', *New England Journal of Medicine*, 387(3):205–16. Available at: https://www.nejm.org/doi/full/10.1056/NEJMoa2206038

25. Reuters (2024) 'Weight-loss drug forecasts jump to $150 billion as supply grows'. Available at: https://www.reuters.com/business/healthcare-pharmaceuticals/weight-loss-drug-forecasts-jump-150-billion-supply-grows-2024-05-28/

26. Jastreboff, A.M., Kaplan, L.M., Frías, J.P., *et al.* (2023) 'Triple–hormone-receptor agonist retatrutide for obesity—a phase 2 trial', *New England Journal of* Medicine, 389(6):514–526. Available at: https://www.nejm.org/doi/full/10.1056/NEJMoa2301972

27. PR Newswire (2024) 'Amgen announces robust weight loss with MariTide in people living with obesity or overweight at 52 weeks in a phase 2 study'. Available at: https://www.prnewswire.com/news-releases/amgen-announces-robust-weight-loss-with-maritide-in-people-living-with-obesity-or-overweight-at-52-weeks-in-a-phase-2-study-302316464.html

28. Melson, E., Ashraf, U., Papamargaritis, D., *et al.* (2024) 'What is the pipeline for future medications for obesity?', *Int J Obes* (2024). https://doi.org/10.1038/s41366-024-01473-y. Available at: https://www.nature.com/articles/s41366-024-01473-y#Sec2

29. Knop, Filip K., Aroda, V.R., do Vale, R.D., *et al.* ( 2023) 'Oral semaglutide 50mg taken once per day in adults with overweight or obesity (OASIS 1): a randomised, double-blind, placebo-controlled, phase 3 trial', *The Lancet*, 402(10403): 705 – 719. Available at: https://www.thelancet.com/journals/lancet/article/PIIS0140-6736(23)01185-6/abstract

## Chapter 5: How the Weight Loss Medications Work

1. Gearhardt, A.N, Bueno, N.B., DiFeliceantonio, A.G., *et al*. (2023) 'Social, clinical, and policy implications of ultra-processed food addiction', *BMJ* 2023;383:e075354. Available at: https://www.bmj.com/content/383/bmj-2023-075354

2. Kenny, P.J. (2011) 'Reward Mechanisms in Obesity: New Insights and Future Directions', *Neuron,* 69 (4): 664–79. Available at: https://www.sciencedirect.com/science/article/pii/S0896627311001140

3. DiFeliceantonio A.G., Coppin, G., Rigoux, L., *et al*. (2018) 'Supra-additive effects of combining fat and carbohydrate on food reward', *Cell Metab.*, 28(1):33–44.e3. doi: 10.1016/j.cmet.2018.05.018. Available at: https://pubmed.ncbi.nlm.nih.gov/29909968/
   Hicks, T. (2023) 'Ultra-processed foods may be as addictive as smoking', *Medical News Today*. Available at: https://www.medicalnewstoday.com/articles/ultra-processed-foods-may-be-as-addictive-as-smoking-study-says

4. Weight Watchers (2024) 'WeightWatchers Unveils "Beyond Hunger: Understanding Food Noise" report offering insights into the experience of ongoing, intrusive thoughts about food'. Available at: https://corporate.ww.com/news/news-details/2024/Weight-Watchers-Unveils-Beyond-Hunger-Understanding-Food-Noise-Report-Offering-Insights-Into-the-Experience-of-Ongoing-Intrusive-Thoughts-About-Food/default.aspx

5. *Independent* (2024) 'Richard Osman opens up about his "ever-present" addiction to food'. Available at: https://www.independent.co.uk/arts-entertainment/tv/news/richard-osman-food-addiction-overeating-b2530786.html

6. Gearhardt, A., Bueno, N.B., DiFeliceantonio, A.G., *et al*. (2023) 'Social, clinical, and policy implications of ultra-processed food addiction', *BMJ*, 383:e075354. Available at: https://www.bmj.com/content/383/bmj-2023-075354

7. Yau, Y.H. and Potenza, M.N. (2013) 'Stress and eating behaviors', *Minerva Endocrinol.* 38(3):255–67. Available at: https://pmc.ncbi.nlm.nih.gov/articles/PMC4214609/

8. Yau, Y.H. and Potenza, M.N. (2013) 'Stress and eating behaviors', *Minerva Endocrinol.* 38(3):255–67. Available at: https://pmc.ncbi.nlm.nih.gov/articles/PMC4214609/

9. Hayes, M.R. and Schmidt, H.D. (2016) 'GLP-1 influences food and drug reward', Current Opinion in Behavioral Sciences, 9: 66–70, https://doi.org/10.1016/j.cobeha.2016.02.005. Available at: https://www.sciencedirect.com/science/article/pii/S2352154616300274

10. Edvardsson, C.E., Vestlund, J., Ericson, M. Jerlhag, E. (2024) 'The GLP-1 receptor agonist exendin-4 reduces taurine and glycine in nucleus accumbens of male rats, an effect tentatively involving the nucleus tractus solitarius', *Frontiers Pharmacology*, 15,

https://doi.org/10.3389/fphar.2024.1439203. Available at: https://www.frontiersin.org/journals/pharmacology/articles/10.3389/fphar.2024.1439203/full?utm_source=chatgpt.com

11. Kooij, K. L., IJsbrand Koster, D., Eeltink, E. (2024) 'GLP-1 receptor agonist semaglutide reduces appetite while increasing dopamine reward signaling' *Elsevier, Neuroscience Applied.* Available at: https://www.sciencedirect.com/science/article/pii/S2772408523029071#bib5

12. *ScienceDirect* (n.d.) 'Incretin – an overview'. Available at: https://www.sciencedirect.com/topics/medicine-and-dentistry/incretin

13. Klausen, M.K., Thomsen, M., Wortwein, G. and Fink-Jensen, A. (2022) 'The role of glucagon-like peptide 1 (GLP-1) in addictive disorders', *British Journal of Pharmacology*, 179(4),625–641. https://doi.org/10.1111/bph.15677. Available at: https://bpspubs.onlinelibrary.wiley.com/doi/10.1111/bph.15677

14. Edvardsson, C.E., Vestlund, J., Ericson, M. Jerlhag, E. (2024) 'The GLP-1 receptor agonist exendin-4 reduces taurine and glycine in nucleus accumbens of male rats, an effect tentatively involving the nucleus tractus solitarius', *Frontiers Pharmacology*, 15, https://doi.org/10.3389/fphar.2024.1439203 Available at: https://www.frontiersin.org/journals/pharmacology/articles/10.3389/fphar.2024.1439203/full?utm_source=chatgpt.com

15. Van Bloemendaal, L., Veltman, D. J., Ten Kulve, J. S., Groot, P. F. C., *et al.* (2015) 'Brain reward-system activation in response to anticipation and consumption of palatable food is altered by glucagon-like peptide-1 receptor activation in humans', Sep;17(9):878–86. doi: 10.1111/dom.12506. *PubMed*. Available at: https://pubmed.ncbi.nlm.nih.gov/26094857/

16. Shah, M. and Vella, A. (2014) 'Effects of GLP-1 on appetite and weight', *Rev Endocr Metab Disord.* 15(3):181–7. doi: 10.1007/s11154-014-9289-5. Available at: https://pmc.ncbi.nlm.nih.gov/articles/PMC4119845/

17. Müller, T.D., Finan, B., Bloom, S.R., *et al.* (2019) 'Glucagon-like peptide 1 (GLP-1)', *Molecular Metabolism*, 30: 72–130. https://doi.org/10.1016/j.molmet.2019.09.010. Available at: https://www.sciencedirect.com/science/article/pii/S2212877819309135#bib685

    Schlögl, H., Kabisch, S., Horstmann, A., *et al.* (2013) 'Exenatide-induced reduction in energy intake is associated with increase in hypothalamic connectivity', *Diabetes Care*, 36(7):1933–40. doi: 10.2337/dc12-1925. Available at: https://pubmed.ncbi.nlm.nih.gov/23462665/DC121925 1933..1940 (silverchair.com)

18. Bu, T., Sun, Z., Pan, Y., *et al.* (2024) 'Glucagon-like peptide-1: new regulator in lipid metabolism', *Diabetes Metab J.*, 48(3):354–372. doi: 10.4093/dmj.2023.0277. Available at:

https://pubmed.ncbi.nlm.nih.gov/38650100/#:~:text=In%20recent%20years%2C%20 basic%20and,metabolism%2C%20and%20promoting%20adipose%20browning.

19. Maselli, D.B. and Camilleri, M. (2021) 'Effects of GLP-1 and Its analogs on gastric physiology in diabetes mellitus and obesity', *Adv Exp Med Biol.*, 1307:171–192. doi: 10.1007/5584_2020_496. Available at: https://pubmed.ncbi.nlm.nih.gov/32077010/

20. Holst, J.J. (2019) 'The incretin system in healthy humans: the role of GIP and GLP-1', *Metabolism*, 96: 46–55, https://doi.org/10.1016/j.metabol.2019.04.014. Available at: https://www.sciencedirect.com/science/article/pii/S0026049519300861

## Chapter 6: Side Effects and Risks

1. *Mirror* online (2024) 'Stephen Fry warns about dangers of "fat jabs" like Ozempic after drastic 5st weight-loss and vomit hell', 20 March. Available at: https://www.mirror.co.uk/3am/celebrity-news/stephen-fry-issues-stark-warning-32401925

2. *Daily Mail* (2023) 'Boris Johnson: The wonder drug I hoped would stop my 11.30pm fridge raids for cheddar and chorizo didn't work for me. But I still believe it could change the lives of millions', 16 June. Available at: https://www.dailymail.co.uk/news/article-12203407/BORIS-JOHNSON-Wonder-drug-hoped-stop-raids-cheddar-chorizo-didnt-work-me.html

3. NIH (2021) STEP 1: Research Study Investigating How Well Semaglutide Works in People Suffering From Overweight or Obesity (STEP 1) Available at: https://clinicaltrials.gov/study/NCT03548935?tab=results

   Wharton, S., Calanna, S., Davies, M., *et al.* (2021) 'Gastrointestinal tolerability of once-weekly semaglutide 2.4mg in adults with overweight or obesity, and the relationship between gastrointestinal adverse events and weight loss', *Diabetes, Obesity and Metabolism*, 24(1):94–105. Available at: https://dom-pubs.onlinelibrary.wiley.com/doi/full/10.1111/dom.14551

4. *Daily Mail* (2024) 'Sharon Osbourne, 72, tries to go incognito on LA outing amid fears about her weight loss', 9 December. Available at: https://www.dailymail.co.uk/tvshowbiz/article-14175125/sharon-osbourne-incognito-la-weight-loss.html

   *Daily Mail* (2023) 'Sharon Osbourne opens up about Russell Brand, her shocking weight loss – and her stormy marriage: Why I turned a blind eye to Ozzy's groupies', 17 November. Available at: https://www.dailymail.co.uk/femail/article-12747755/Sharon-Osbourne-opens-Russell-Brand-shocking-weight-loss-stormy-marriage-turned-blind-eye-Ozzys-groupies.html

5. Reuters (2018) 'Weight-loss surgery tied to increases in divorces, marriages'. Available at: https://www.reuters.com/article/business/healthcare-pharmaceuticals/weight-loss-surgery-tied-to-increases-in-divorces-marriages-idUSKCN1HA2G5/#:~:text=Among%20patients%20who%20were%20married,percent%20in%20the%20other%20group.

   *Guardian* (2019) 'Bariatric divorce: why extreme weight loss leads to break ups' 17 June. Available at: https://www.theguardian.com/lifeandstyle/2019/jun/17/bariatric-divorce-why-extreme-weight-loss-leads-to-break-ups

6. Wadden, T., Brown, G.K., Egebjerg, C. (2024) 'Psychiatric safety of semaglutide for weight management in people without known major psychopathology: post hoc analysis of the STEP 1, 2, 3, and 5 trials', *Psychiatry and Behavioral Health, JAMA Intern Med.*, 184(11):1290–1300. doi:10.1001/jamainternmed.2024.4346. Available at: https://jamanetwork.com/journals/jamainternalmedicine/fullarticle/2823084

7. NIH (2024) 'Semaglutide associated with lower risk of suicidal ideations compared to other treatments prescribed for obesity or type 2 diabetes'. Available at: https://www.nih.gov/news-events/news-releases/glutide-associated-lower-risk-suicidal-ideations-compared-other-treatments-prescribed-obesity-or-type-2-diabetes#:~:text=Semaglutide%2C%20a%20highly%20popular%20medication,2%20diabetes%20that%20work%20via

8. Van Gennip, A.C.E., Schram, M.T., Kohler, S., *et al.* (2023) 'Association of type 2 diabetes according to the number of risk factors within the recommended range with incidence of major depression and clinically relevant depressive symptoms: a prospective analysis', 4(2): E63–E71. Available at: https://www.thelancet.com/journals/lanhl/article/PIIS2666-7568(22)00291-4/fulltext#:~:text=Major%20depression%20is%20increasingly%20recognised,Skinner%2C%20TC%20%E2%88%99%20et%20al.

9. Nathani, P., Desai, M., Patel, H.K., *et al.* (2024) 'Incidence of gastrointestinal side effects in patients prescribed glucagon-like peptide-1 (GLP-1) analogs: real-world evidence', Digestive Disease Week ePoster Library. Available at: https://eposters.ddw.org/ddw/2024/ddw-2024/414874/piyush.nathani.incidence.of.gastrointestinal.side.effects.in.patients.html?f=listing%3D0%2Abrowseby%3D8%2Asortby%3D1%2Asearch%3Dsa1964

10. Lu, J., Liu, H., Zhou, Q., *et al.* (2023) 'A potentially serious adverse effect of GLP-1 receptor agonists', Acta Pharm Sin B., 13(5):2291–2293. doi: 10.1016/j.apsb.2023.02.020. Available at: https://pmc.ncbi.nlm.nih.gov/articles/PMC10213739/#:~:text=Dapiglutide%20was%20shown%20to%20dose,SBS)%20and%20intestinal%20failure10.

11. Gudin, B., Ladhari, C., Robin, P. (2020), *et al*. 'Incretin-based drugs and intestinal obstruction: a pharmacovigilance study', *Therapie*, 75(6):641–647. doi: 10.1016/j.therap.2020.02.024. Available at: https://pubmed.ncbi.nlm.nih.gov/32418731/

12. Faillie, J.L., Yin, H., Yu O.H.Y., *et al*. (2022) 'Incretin-based drugs and risk of intestinal obstruction among patients with type 2 diabetes', *Clin Pharmacol Ther.,* 111(1):272–282. doi: 10.1002/cpt.2430. Available at: https://pubmed.ncbi.nlm.nih.gov/34587280/

13. BBC (2024) 'Nurse's death linked to weight-loss drug Mounjaro approved on NHS', 8 November. Available at: https://www.bbc.co.uk/news/articles/cz6jg6nw2zeo

14. Lilly 'What is the incidence of pancreatitis associated with Zepbound™ (tirzepatide)?'. Available at: https://medical.lilly.com/us/products/answers/what-is-the-incidence-of-pancreatitis-associated-with-zepbound-tirzepatide-209516# reference-f355d332-b75f-44ac-a33b-5e47a60e4026-3

15. Nreu, B., Dicembrini, I., Tinti, F., *et al*. (2023) 'Pancreatitis and pancreatic cancer in patients with type 2 diabetes treated with glucagon-like peptide-1 receptor agonists: an updated meta-analysis of randomized controlled trials', *Minerva Endocrinol (Torino),* 48(2):206–213. doi: 10.23736/S2724-6507.20.03219-8. Available at: https://pubmed.ncbi.nlm.nih.gov/32720500/

16. Masson, W., Lobo, M., Barbagelata, L., *et al*. (2024) 'Acute pancreatitis due to different semaglutide regimens: an updated meta-analysis', *Endocrinología, Diabetes y Nutrición*, 71(3): 124–132, https://doi.org/10.1016/j.endinu.2024.01.001. Available at: https://www.sciencedirect.com/science/article/abs/pii/S253001642400020X

17. Sodhi, M., Rezaeianzadeh, R., Kezouh, A., *et al*. (2023) 'Risk of gastrointestinal adverse events associated with glucagon-like peptide-1 receptor agonists for weight loss', *JAMA*, 330(18):1795–1797. doi:10.1001/jama.2023.19574. Available at: https://jamanetwork.com/journals/jama/fullarticle/2810542

18. A 2022 review in the journal *JAMA Internal Medicine* found GLP1s were associated with a 27% greater risk of gallstones

19. Erlinger, S. (2000) 'Gallstones in obesity and weight loss', *European Journal of Gastroenterology & Hepatology*, 12(12):1347–1352. Available at: https://journals.lww.com/eurojgh/abstract/2000/12120/gallstones_in_obesity_and_weight_loss.15.aspx

20. Silverii, G.A., Monami, M., Gallo, M., *et al*. (2024) 'Glucagon-like peptide-1 receptor agonists and risk of thyroid cancer: a systematic review and meta-analysis of randomized controlled trials', *Diabetes Obes Metab.*, 26(3):891–900. doi: 10.1111/dom.15382. Available at: https://pubmed.ncbi.nlm.nih.gov/38018310/

Hu, W., Song, R., Cheng, R., *et al.* (2022) 'Use of GLP-1 receptor agonists and occurrence of thyroid disorders: a meta-analysis of randomized controlled trials', *Frontiers Endocrinology*, 13, https://doi.org/10.3389/fendo.2022.927859. Available at: https://www.frontiersin.org/journals/endocrinology/articles/10.3389/fendo.2022.927859/full

ASCO Post (2024) 'new findings suggest no correlation between glp-1 receptor agonists and thyroid cancer risk. Available at: https://ascopost.com/news/april-2024/new-findings-suggest-no-correlation-between-glp-1-receptor-agonists-and-thyroid-cancer-risk/

## Chapter 7: Health Benefits of the Jabs Outside of Weight Loss

1. Zhao, X., Wang, M., Wen, Z., *et al.* (2021) 'GLP-1 receptor agonists: beyond their pancreatic effects', *Front Endocrinol (Lausanne)*, 12:721135. doi: 10.3389/fendo.2021.721135. Available at: https://pmc.ncbi.nlm.nih.gov/articles/PMC8419463/

2. Bendotti, G., Montefusco, L., Lunati, M.E., *et al.* (2022) 'The anti-inflammatory and immunological properties of GLP-1 receptor agonists', *Pharmacological Research*, 182, https://doi.org/10.1016/j.phrs.2022.106320. Available at: https://www.sciencedirect.com/science/article/pii/S1043661822002651

   *New Scientist* (2024) 'The surprising mental health and brain benefits of weight-loss drugs' Available at: https://www.newscientist.com/article/mg26234953-900-the-surprising-mental-health-and-brain-benefits-of-weight-loss-drugs/

3. Ferrucci, L. and Fabbri, E. (2018) 'Inflammageing: chronic inflammation in ageing, cardiovascular disease, and frailty', *Nat Rev Cardiol.*, 15(9):505–522. doi: 10.1038/s41569-018-0064-2. Available at: https://pmc.ncbi.nlm.nih.gov/articles/PMC6146930/#:~:text=On%20the%20basis%20of%20these,the%20biology%20of%20ageing20.

4. Pang, J., Feng, J.N., Ling, W. and Jin, T. (2022) 'The anti-inflammatory feature of glucagon-like peptide-1 and its based diabetes drugs – Therapeutic potential exploration in lung injury', *Acta Pharm Sin B.*, 12(11):4040–4055. doi: 10.1016/j.apsb.2022.06.003. Available at: https://pmc.ncbi.nlm.nih.gov/articles/PMC9643154/

5. Wong, C.K., McLean, B.A., Baggio, L.L., *et al.* (2024) 'Central glucagon-like peptide 1 receptor activation inhibits toll-like receptor agonist-induced inflammation', *Cell Metab.*, 36(1):130–143.e5. doi: 10.1016/j.cmet.2023.11.009. Available at: https://pubmed.ncbi.nlm.nih.gov/38113888/

6. Lincoff, A.M., Brown-Frandsen, K., Colhoun, H.M. *et al.* (2023) 'Semaglutide and cardiovascular outcomes in obesity without diabetes', *New England Journal of Medicine*, 389(24). Available at https://www.nejm.org/doi/full/10.1056/NEJMoa2307563

   British Heart Foundation (2024) 'Weight loss drugs could have cardiovascular benefits, new research shows'. Available at: https://www.bhf.org.uk/what-we-do/news-from-the-bhf/news-archive/2024/may/weight-loss-drugs-could-have-cardiovascular-benefits-new-research-shows

   UCL News (2024) 'Weight loss drug semaglutide linked to better heart health'. Available at: https://www.ucl.ac.uk/news/2024/may/weight-loss-drug-semaglutide-linked-better-heart-health#:~:text=The%20weight%20loss%20drug%20semaglutide,a%20UCL%2Dled%20research%20team.

7. Perkovic, V., Tuttle, K.R., Rossing P., *et al.* (2024) 'Effects of Semaglutide on Chronic Kidney Disease in Patients with Type 2 Diabetes' *New England Journal of Medicine.* Available at: https://www.nejm.org/doi/full/10.1056/NEJMoa2403347

8. Ma, Y., Ajnakina, O., Steptoe, A. (2020) 'Higher risk of dementia in English older individuals who are overweight or obese', *International Journal of Epidemiology*, 49(4): 1353–1365, https://doi.org/10.1093/ije/dyaa099 Available at: https://academic.oup.com/ije/article/49/4/1353/5861491

9. Aviles-Olmos, I., Dickson, J., Kefalopoulou, Z., *et al.* (2013) 'Exenatide and the treatment of patients with Parkinson's disease' *Journal of Clinical Investigation.* Available at: https://pmc.ncbi.nlm.nih.gov/articles/PMC3668846/

10. Wang, L., Wang, W., Kaelber, D.C., *et al.* (2024) 'GLP-1 receptor agonists and colorectal cancer risk in drug-naive patients with type 2 diabetes, with and without overweight/obesity', *JAMA Oncol.,* 10(2):256–258. doi:10.1001/jamaoncol.2023.5573. Available at: https://jamanetwork.com/journals/jamaoncology/fullarticle/2812769

11. BBC Future ' "These are people in the prime of life": The worrying puzzle behind the rise in early-onset cancer'. Available at: https://www.bbc.com/future/article/20241004-the-puzzle-of-rising-early-onset-breast-and-colorectal-cancer-in-younger-people

12. Chuong, V., Farokhnia, M., Khom, S., *et al.* (2023) 'The glucagon-like peptide-1 (GLP-1) analogue semaglutide reduces alcohol drinking and modulates central GABA neurotransmission', JCI Insight. Available at: https://insight.jci.org/articles/view/170671#:~:text=Administration%20of%20GLP%2D1%20itself,alcohol%20(6%2C%2017)

   Klausen, M.K., Thomsen, M., Wortwein, G., and Fink-Jensen, A. (2022) 'The role of glucagon-like peptide 1 (GLP-1) in addictive disorders', *Br J Pharmacol.*, 179(4):

625–641. doi: 10.1111/bph.15677. Available at: https://pubmed.ncbi.nlm.nih.gov/34532853/

Badulescu, S., Tabassum, A., Han Le, G., *et al.* (2024) 'Glucagon-like peptide 1 agonist and effects on reward behaviour: a systematic review', *Physiology & Behavior*, 283, https://doi.org/10.1016/j.physbeh.2024.114622. Available at: (https://www.sciencedirect.com/science/article/pii/S0031938424001677)

13. *Independent* (2017) 'Giving your child a smartphone is like giving them a gram of cocaine, says top addiction expert', 7 June. Available at: https://www.independent.co.uk/news/education/education-news/child-smart-phones-cocaine-addiction-expert-mandy-saligari-harley-street-charter-clinic-technology-teenagers-a7777941.html

14. Meng, S.Q., Cheng, J.L., Li, Y.Y., *et al.* (2022) 'Global prevalence of digital addiction in general population: A systematic review and meta-analysis', *Clin Psychol Rev.*, 92: 102128. doi: 10.1016/j.cpr.2022.102128. Available at: https://pubmed.ncbi.nlm.nih.gov/35150965/

15. Bliddal, H., Bays, H., Czernichow, S., *et al.* (2024) 'STEP 9 Study Group. once-weekly semaglutide in persons with obesity and knee osteoarthritis', *N Engl J Med.*, 391(17): 1573–1583. doi: 10.1056/NEJMoa2403664. Available at: https://pubmed.ncbi.nlm.nih.gov/39476339/

16. Zhu, H., Zhou, L., Wang, Q., *et al.* (2023) 'Glucagon-like peptide-1 receptor agonists as a disease-modifying therapy for knee osteoarthritis mediated by weight loss: findings from the Shanghai Osteoarthritis Cohort', *Ann Rheum Dis.*,82(9):1218–1226. doi: 10.1136/ard-2023-223845. Available at: https://pubmed.ncbi.nlm.nih.gov/37258065/

17. Miller, A., Joyce, B., Bartlet, K.B., and Deckert, J. 'Most GLP-1 Medications Correlated with a Lower Likelihood of Anxiety and Depression Diagnoses'. Available at: https://www.epicresearch.org/articles/most-glp-1-medications-correlated-with-a-lower-likelihood-of-anxiety-and-depression-diagnoses

18. Lechat, B., Naikm G., Reynolds, A., *et al.* (2022) 'Multinight prevalence, variability, and diagnostic misclassification of obstructive sleep apnea', *Am J Respir Crit Care Med.*, 205(5):563–569. doi: 10.1164/rccm.202107-1761OC. Available at: https://pubmed.ncbi.nlm.nih.gov/34904935/

19. Meyer, E.J. and Wittert, G.A. (2024) 'Approach the patient with obstructive sleep apnea and obesity', *The Journal of Clinical Endocrinology & Metabolism*, 109(3): e1267–e1279, https://doi.org/10.1210/clinem/dgad572. Available at: https://academic.oup.com/jcem/article/109/3/e1267/7284057

Kansanen, M., Vanninen, E., Tuunainen, A., *et al.* (1998) 'The effect of a very low-calorie diet-induced weight loss on the severity of obstructive sleep apnoea and autonomic nervous function in obese patients with obstructive sleep apnoea syndrome', *Clin Physiol.*, 18(4):377–85. doi: 10.1046/j.1365-2281.1998.00114.x. Available at: https://pubmed.ncbi.nlm.nih.gov/9715765/

20. Lilly Investors (2024) 'Lilly's tirzepatide was superior to placebo for MASH resolution, and more than half of patients achieved improvement in fibrosis at 52 weeks'. Available at: https://investor.lilly.com/news-releases/news-release-details/lillys-tirzepatide-was-superior-placebo-mash-resolution-and-more

## Chapter 8: How to Use Weight Loss Drugs Safely

1. Obesity Health Alliance (2024) 'Treatment of Overweight and Obesity Position Statement & Evidence Review'. Available at: chrome-extension://efaidnbmnnnibpcaj pcglclefindmkaj/https://obesityhealthalliance.org.uk/wp-content/uploads/2024/10/OHA_Treatment_2024.pdf

2. Rehman, A. and Nashwan, A.J. (2024) 'The rising threat of counterfeit GLP-1 receptor agonists: Implications for public health', *Journal of Medicine, Surgery, and Public Health*, 3, https://doi.org/10.1016/j.glmedi.2024.100136. Available at: https://www.sciencedirect.com/science/article/pii/S2949916X24000896

3. UK Government (2023) 'Falsified Ozempic (semaglutide) pens identified at two wholesalers in the UK'. Available at: https://www.gov.uk/government/news/falsified-ozempic-semaglutide-pens-identified-at-two-wholesalers-in-the-uk

4. Eli Lilly and Company Vs Pivotal Peptides LLC. Available at: https://cdn.arstechnica.net/wp-content/uploads/2024/10/0001.00_2024-10-21-Complaint-for-False-Advertising-and-Promotion-Pivotal-1.pdf

5. Wilding, J.P.H., Batterham, R.L., Davies, M., *et al.* 'Weight regain and cardiometabolic effects after withdrawal of semaglutide: The STEP 1 trial extension', *Diabetes, Obesity and Metabolism*. Available at: https://discovery.ucl.ac.uk/id/eprint/10149199/1/Diabetes%20Obesity%20Metabolism%20-%202022%20-%20Wilding%20-%20Weight%20regain%20and%20cardiometabolic%20effects%20after%20withdrawal%20of%20semaglutide%20.pdf

6. Aronne, L.J., Sattar, N., Horn, D.B., *et al.* (2024) 'SURMOUNT-4 Investigators. Continued Treatment with Tirzepatide for Maintenance of Weight Reduction in Adults With Obesity: The SURMOUNT-4 Randomized Clinical Trial', *JAMA*, 331(1):

38–48. doi: 10.1001/jama.2023.24945. Available at: https://pmc.ncbi.nlm.nih.gov/articles/PMC10714284/

7.  Rubino, D., Abrahamsson, N. and Davies, M.D., *et al.* (2021) 'Effect of continued weekly subcutaneous semaglutide vs placebo on weight loss maintenance in adults with overweight or obesity: The STEP 4 Randomized Clinical Trial', *Clinical Pharmacy and Pharmacology* | JAMA, 325(14):1414–1425. doi:10.1001/jama.2021.3224. Available at: https://jamanetwork.com/journals/jama/fullarticle/2777886

8.  Reuters (2024) 'Exclusive: Most patients stop using Wegovy, Ozempic for weight loss within two years'. Available at: https://www.reuters.com/business/healthcare-pharmaceuticals/most-patients-stop-using-wegovy-ozempic-weight-loss-within-two-years-analysis-2024-07-10/#:~:text=For%20Wegovy%2C%2024.1%25%20of%20patients,co%2Dauthor%20of%20the%20analysis.&text=Both%20Novo%20and%20Lilly%20have,demand%20for%20the%20new%20medicines.

9.  BBC Future (2024) 'What happens when you stop taking weight-loss drugs?'. Available at: https://www.bbc.com/future/article/20240521-what-happens-when-you-stop-taking-ozempic

10. *The Times* (2024) 'I tried Ozempic microdosing, the secret way the rich lose weight' 17 December. Available at: https://www.thetimes.com/article/a6e0f8c4-a407-4fc7-a781-d6966cba9a3a

11. NBC (2024) 'Kate Moss' sister shares story of "scary" hospitalization after Ozempic overdose', 12 September. Available at: https://www.nbcconnecticut.com/entertainment/entertainment-news/kate-moss-sister-shares-story-of-scary-hospitalization-after-ozempic-overdose/3384724/?os=av&ref=app

## Chapter 9: Staying Nourished – How to Eat Well On and Off the Weight Loss Drugs

1.  Estruch, R., Ros, E., Salas-Salvado, J., *et al.* (2018) 'Primary Prevention of Cardiovascular Disease with a Mediterranean Diet Supplemented with Extra-Virgin Olive Oil or Nuts', *New England Journal of Medicine*, 378(25). Available at: https://www.nejm.org/doi/full/10.1056/NEJMoa1800389

2.  Jacka, F.N., O'Neil, A., Opie, R., *et al.* (2017) 'A randomised controlled trial of dietary improvement for adults with major depression (the 'SMILES' trial)', BMC Medicine, 15: 23. Available at: https://bmcmedicine.biomedcentral.com/articles/10.1186/s12916-017-0791-y#Sec2

3. Radkhah, N., Rasouli, A., Majnouni, A., *et al.* (2023) 'The effect of Mediterranean diet instructions on depression, anxiety, stress, and anthropometric indices: A randomized, double-blind, controlled clinical trial', *Prev Med Rep.*, 36:102469. doi: 10.1016/j. Available at: https://pmc.ncbi.nlm.nih.gov/articles/PMC10587518/

4. Buettner, D. *Blue Zones* (n.d.) 'Sardinia, Italy'. Available at: https://www.bluezones.com/explorations/sardinia-italy/

5. *Guardian* (2022) '"I've lived through hunger and war": tiny Italian town sets record as 10th resident turns 100', 14 February. Available at: https://www.theguardian.com/world/2022/feb/14/10-residents-over-100-record-breaking-sardinia-town-perdasdefogu

6. Wang, C., Murgia, M.A., Baptista, J., *et al.* (2022) 'Sardinian dietary analysis for longevity: a review of the literature', *J. Ethn. Food* 9, 33. https://doi.org/10.1186/s42779-022-00152-5 Available at: https://journalofethnicfoods.biomedcentral.com/articles/10.1186/s42779-022-00152-5#citeas

7. Oregon State University (2005) 'Flavonoid-rich foods (FRF): A promising nutraceutical approach against lifespan-shortening diseases – PMC'. Available at: https://lpi.oregonstate.edu/mic/dietary-factors/phytochemicals/flavonoids#:~:text=Biological%20activities%20related%20to%20the,occurring%20during%20atherogenesis%20(43).

8. Spencer, N.J., and Hu, H. (2020) 'Enteric nervous system: sensory transduction, neural circuits and gastrointestinal motility', *Nat Rev Gastroenterol Hepatol.*, 17(6):338–351. doi: 10.1038/s41575-020-0271-2. Available at: https://pubmed.ncbi.nlm.nih.gov/32152479/

   Carabotti, M, Scirocco, A., Maselli, M.A. and Severi, C. (2015) 'The gut-brain axis: interactions between enteric microbiota, central and enteric nervous systems', *Ann Gastroenterol.*, 28(2):203–209. Available at: https://pmc.ncbi.nlm.nih.gov/articles/PMC4367209/

9. Dehghan, M., Mente, A., Rangarajan, S., *et al.* (2018) 'Association of dairy intake with cardiovascular disease and mortality in 21 countries from five continents (PURE): a prospective cohort study', *The Lancet*, 392 (10161): p2288–97. Available at: https://www.thelancet.com/journals/lancet/article/PIIS0140-6736(18)31812-9/abstract

10. Astrup, A., Geiker, N.R.W., and Magkos, F. (2019) 'Effects of Full-Fat and Fermented Dairy Products on Cardiometabolic Disease: Food Is More Than the Sum of Its Parts', *Adv Nutr.*, 10(5):924S–930S. doi: 10.1093/advances/nmz069. Available at: https://pmc.ncbi.nlm.nih.gov/articles/PMC6743821/

11. Hibbeln, J.R., Spiller, P., and Brenna, T. (2019) 'Relationships between seafood consumption during pregnancy and childhood and neurocognitive development: Two systematic reviews', *Prostaglandins, Leukotrienes and Essential Fatty Acids*, 151: 14–36, https://doi.org/10.1016/j.plefa.2019.10.002. Available at: https://www.sciencedirect.com/science/article/pii/S0952327819301929

12. Lund University (2018) 'Fish accounted for surprisingly large part of the Stone Age diet'. Available at: https://www.lunduniversity.lu.se/article/fish-accounted-surprisingly-large-part-stone-age-diet

    *Science Daily* (2018) 'Fish accounted for surprisingly large part of the Stone Age diet'. Available at: https://www.sciencedaily.com/releases/2018/03/180319120536.htm

    Challa, H.J., Bandlamudi, M., and Uppaluri, K.R. (2023) 'Paleolithic Diet'. In: StatPearls. Treasure Island (FL): StatPearls Publishing; 2025 Jan. Available from: https://www.ncbi.nlm.nih.gov/books/NBK482457/

## Chapter 10: How to Protect Your Muscles

1. Jastreboff, A.M., Aronne, L.J., Ahmad, N.N., *et al.* (2022) 'Tirzepatide once weekly for the treatment of obesity', *New England Journal of Medicine*, 387(3): 387:205–216, DOI: 10.1056/NEJMoa2206038. Available at: https://www.nejm.org/doi/full/10.1056/NEJMoa2206038

2. Kim, J.E., O'Connor, L.E., Sands, L.P., *et al.* (2106) 'Effects of dietary protein intake on body composition changes after weight loss in older adults: a systematic review and meta-analysis', *Nutr Rev.*, 74(3):210–24. doi: 10.1093/nutrit/nuv065. Available at: https://pmc.ncbi.nlm.nih.gov/articles/PMC4892287/

3. Martinez-Cordero, C., Kuzawa, C.W., Sloboda, D.M., *et al.* (2012) 'Testing the Protein Leverage Hypothesis in a free-living human population', *Appetite*, 59(2): 312–315, https://doi.org/10.1016/j.appet.2012.05.013. Available at: https://www.sciencedirect.com/science/article/abs/pii/S0195666312001699?via%3Dihub

    Raubenheimer, D. and Simpson, S.J. (2023) 'Protein appetite as an integrator in the obesity system: the protein leverage hypothesis', *Philosophical Transactions of the Royal Society B: Biological Sciences*. Available at: https://royalsocietypublishing.org/doi/10.1098/rstb.2022.0212

4. Frimel, T.N., Sinacore, D.R. and Villareal, D.T. (2008) 'Exercise attenuates the weight-loss-induced reduction in muscle mass in frail obese older adults', *Med Sci Sports Exerc.*,

40(7):1213–9. doi: 10.1249/MSS.0b013e31816a85ce. Available at: https://pmc.ncbi.nlm.nih.gov/articles/PMC2650077/

Ballor, D.L., Katch, V.L., Becque, M.D. and Marks, C.R. (1988) 'Resistance weight training during caloric restriction enhances lean body weight maintenance', *American Journal of Clinical Nutrition*, 47 (1): 19–25, https://doi.org/10.1093/ajcn/47.1.19. Available at: https://www.sciencedirect.com/science/article/abs/pii/S0002916523165981

5. Fielding, R.A. (1995) 'The role of progressive resistance training and nutrition in the preservation of lean body mass in the elderly', *Journal of the American College of Nutrition*, *14*(6), 587–594. https://doi.org/10.1080/07315724.1995.10718547. Available at: https://www.tandfonline.com/doi/abs/10.1080/07315724.1995.10718547

6. Nasri Marzuca-Nassr, G., Alegría-Molina, A., SanMartín-Calísto, Y., *et al.* (2023) 'Muscle mass and strength gains following resistance exercise training in older adults 65–75 years and older adults above 85 years', *International Journal of Sport Nutrition and Exercise Metabolism*, 34(1). Available at: https://journals.humankinetics.com/view/journals/ijsnem/34/1/article-p11.xml

7. Lopez, P., Taaffe, D.R., Galvão, D.A., *et al.* (2022) 'Resistance training effectiveness on body composition and body weight outcomes in individuals with overweight and obesity across the lifespan: A systematic review and meta-analysis', *Obes Rev.,* 23(5):e13428. doi: 10.1111/obr.13428. Available at: https://pubmed.ncbi.nlm.nih.gov/35191588/

8. Momma, H., Kawakami, R., Honda, T., *et al.* (2022) 'Muscle-strengthening activities are associated with lower risk and mortality in major non-communicable diseases: a systematic review and meta-analysis of cohort studies', *Br J Sports Med.,* 56(13):755–763. doi: 10.1136/bjsports-2021-105061. Available at: https://pubmed.ncbi.nlm.nih.gov/35228201/

9. Steven, S., Hollingsworth, K. G., Al-Mrabeh, A. *et al.* (2016) 'Very Low-Calorie Diet and 6 Months of Weight Stability in Type 2 Diabetes: Pathophysiological Changes in Responders and Nonresponders' *PubMed.* Available at: https://pubmed.ncbi.nlm.nih.gov/27002059/

10. Erickson, K.I., Voss, M.W., Prakash, R.S., *et al.* (2011) 'Exercise training increases size of hippocampus and improves memory', *PNAS*, 108 (7) 3017–3022. Available at: https://www.pnas.org/doi/full/10.1073/pnas.1015950108

11. Defina, L.F., Willis, B.L., Radford, N.B., *et al.* (2013) 'The association between midlife cardiorespiratory fitness levels and later-life dementia: a cohort study', *Ann Intern Med.,* 158(3):162–8. doi: 10.7326/0003-4819-158-3-201302050-00005. Available at: https://pubmed.ncbi.nlm.nih.gov/23381040/

12. Spiegelhalter, D. (2012) 'Using speed of ageing and "microlives" to communicate the effects of lifetime habits and environment', *BMJ*, 345 doi: https://doi.org/10.1136/bmj.e8223. Available at: https://www.bmj.com/content/345/bmj.e8223

13. Lee, D.H., Rezende, L.F.M., Joh, H.K., *et al.* (2022) 'Long-term leisure-time physical activity intensity and all-cause and cause-specific mortality: a prospective cohort of US adults', *Circulation*, 146(7):523–534. doi: 10.1161/CIRCULATIONAHA.121.058162. Available at: https://pubmed.ncbi.nlm.nih.gov/35876019/

14. Hong, A.R. and Kim, S.W. (2018) 'Effects of resistance exercise on bone health', *Endocrinol Metab (Seoul)*, 33(4):435–444. doi: 10.3803/EnM.2018.33.4.435. Available at: https://pmc.ncbi.nlm.nih.gov/articles/PMC6279907/

## Chapter 11: The Plan

1. Morris, E., Aveyard, P., Dyson, P., *et al.* (2019) 'A food-based, low-energy, low-carbohydrate diet for people with type 2 diabetes in primary care: A randomized controlled feasibility trial', *Diabetes, Obesity and Metabolism,* 22(4): 512–50. Available at: https://dom-pubs.onlinelibrary.wiley.com/doi/full/10.1111/dom.13915

2. Vikberg, A., Sorlenm N., Branden, L., *et al.* (2019) 'Effects of resistance training on functional strength and muscle mass in 70-year-old individuals with pre-sarcopenia: a randomized controlled trial', *Journal of the American Medical Directors Association*, 20(1): 28–34. Available at: https://www.sciencedirect.com/science/article/pii/S1525861018305024

3. Steven, S., Hollingsworth, K.G., Al-Mrabeh, A., *et al.* (2016) 'Very low-calorie diet and 6 months of weight stability in type 2 diabetes: pathophysiological changes in responders and nonresponders', *Diabetes Care*, 39(5): 808–15. Available at: https://diabetesjournals.org/care/article/39/5/808/30678/Very-Low-Calorie-Diet-and-6-Months-of-Weight

4. Savage, J.S., Hoffman, L. and Birch, L.L. (2009) 'Dieting, restraint, and disinhibition predict women's weight change over 6 y', *American Journal of Clinical Nutrition*, 90(1): 33–40. Available at: https://pubmed.ncbi.nlm.nih.gov/19439461/

5. Prochaska, J. O. and DiClemente, C.C. (1983). 'Stages and processes of self-change of smoking: Toward an integrative model of change', *Journal of Consulting and Clinical Psychology,* 51(3), 390–395. https://doi.org/10.1037/0022-006X.51.3.390. Available at: https://psycnet.apa.org/record/1983-26480-001

6. Cherry, K. (2024) 'The 6 stages of change'. Very Well Mind. Available at: https://www.verywellmind.com/the-stages-of-change-2794868

7.  Kuijer, R.G. and Boyce, J.A (2014) 'Chocolate cake. Guilt or celebration? Associations with healthy eating attitudes, perceived behavioural control, intentions and weight-loss', *Appetite*,74:48–54. doi: 10.1016/j.appet.2013.11.013. Available at: https://pubmed.ncbi.nlm.nih.gov/24275670/

8.  Bogh, A.F., Jensen, S.B.K., Juhl, C.R., *et al.* (2023) 'Insufficient sleep predicts poor weight loss maintenance after 1 year', *Sleep*, ;46(5):zsac295. doi: 10.1093/sleep/zsac295. Available at: https://pmc.ncbi.nlm.nih.gov/articles/PMC10171640/#:~:text=Results,1%2Dyear%20weight%20maintenance%20phase.

## Conclusion

1.  Food, Farming & Countryside Commission (2024) 'Unhealthy food costing UK over £250 bn'. Available at: https://ffcc.co.uk/news-and-press/unhealthy-food-costing-uk-billions#:~:text=New%20analysis%20commissioned%20by%20the,total%20annual%20UK%20healthcare%20spend.

2.  Harvey, J. (2024) 'NHS England proposes phased launch of obesity injection'. *Pf Media*. Available at: https://pf-media.co.uk/news/nhs-england-proposes-phased-launch-of-obesity-injection/#:~:text=A%20range%20of%20community%2Dbased,and%20Care%20Excellence%20(NICE).

3.  National Institute for Health and Care Excellence (NICE) (2024) 'Consultation on NHS England proposals for a phased launch of obesity injection'. Available at: https://www.nice.org.uk/news/articles/consultation-on-nhs-england-proposals-for-a-phased-launch-of-obesity-injection

## Q&A

1.  Nackers, L.M., Ross, K.M. and Perri, M.G. (2010) 'The association between rate of initial weight loss and long-term success in obesity treatment: does slow and steady win the race?', *Int J Behav Med.*, 17(3):161–7. doi: 10.1007/s12529-010-9092-y. Available at: https://pmc.ncbi.nlm.nih.gov/articles/PMC3780395/#:~:text=Those%20who%20lost%20weight%20at,lost%20at%20a%20SLOW%20rate.

2.  Valabhji, J., Gorton, T., Barron, E., *et al.* (2024) 'Early findings from the NHS Type 2 Diabetes Path to Remission Programme: a prospective evaluation of real-world implementation', *The Lancet Diabetes & Endocrinology*, 12(9): P653-663. Available at: https://www.thelancet.com/journals/landia/article/PIIS2213-8587(24)00194-3/fulltext

# INDEX